COPING SUCCESSFULLY WITH PMS

KAREN EVENNETT graduated from University College London in 1983. She worked in academic publishing before training as a journalist at the London College of Printing in 1986. She now specializes in writing about women's health and relationships and her features appear regularly in the weekly magazines *Woman's Own*, *Woman's Realm* and *Bella*. She lives in Surrey and is married with one daughter, Coco.

Overcoming Common Problems Series

For a full list of titles please contact
Sheldon Press, Marylebone Road, London NW1 4DU

The Assertiveness Workbook
A plan for busy women
JOANNA GUTMANN

Birth Over Thirty
SHEILA KITZINGER

Body Language
How to read others' thoughts by their
gestures
ALLAN PEASE

Body Language in Relationships
DAVID COHEN

Calm Down
How to cope with frustration and anger
DR PAUL HAUCK

Changing Course
How to take charge of your career
SUE DYSON AND STEPHEN HOARE

Comfort for Depression
JANET HORWOOD

Coping Successfully with Agoraphobia
DR KENNETH HAMBLY

Coping Successfully with Migraine
SUE DYSON

Coping Successfully with Pain
NEVILLE SHONE

Coping Successfully with Panic Attacks
SHIRLEY TRICKETT

Coping Successfully with Prostate Problems
ROSY REYNOLDS

Coping Successfully with Your Hyperactive Child
DR PAUL CARSON

Coping Successfully with Your Irritable Bowel
ROSEMARY NICOL

Coping Successfully with Your Second Child
FIONA MARSHALL

Coping with Anxiety and Depression
SHIRLEY TRICKETT

Coping with Blushing
DR ROBERT EDELMANN

Coping with Cot Death
SARAH MURPHY

Coping with Depression and Elation
DR PATRICK McKEON

Coping with Strokes
DR TOM SMITH

Coping with Suicide
DR DONALD SCOTT

Coping with Thrush
CAROLINE CLAYTON

Curing Arthritis Diet Book
MARGARET HILLS

Curing Arthritis – The Drug-Free Way
MARGARET HILLS

Curing Arthritis
More ways to a drug-free life
MARGARET HILLS

Curing Coughs, Colds and Flu – The Drug-Free Way
MARGARET HILLS

Curing Illness – The Drug-Free Way
MARGARET HILLS

Depression
DR PAUL HAUCK

Divorce and Separation
Every woman's guide to a new life
ANGELA WILLANS

Don't Blame Me!
How to stop blaming yourself
and other people
TONY GOUGH

Everything You Need to Know about Shingles
DR ROBERT YOUNGSON

Family First Aid and Emergency Handbook
DR ANDREW STANWAY

Overcoming Common Problems Series

Overcoming Common Problems Series

Overcoming Common Problems

COPING SUCCESSFULLY
WITH PMS

Karen Evennett

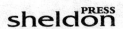

First published in Great Britain in 1995 by
Sheldon Press, SPCK, Marylebone Road, London NW1 4DU

British Library Cataloguing-in-Publication Data
A catalogue record for this book is available from the British Library

ISBN 0–85969–726–6

Photoset by Deltatype Ltd, Ellesmere Port, Cheshire
Printed in Great Britain by Biddles Ltd, Guildford and King's Lynn

Contents

Acknowledgements

My first thanks go to all the women who kindly allowed me to interview them, and without whom this book would not have been possible. I would also like to thank: The National Association for Premenstrual Syndrome (NAPS) and particularly Althea Wheeler, whose long chats on the phone and help in sending out my questionnaire to members were invaluable; Maryon Stewart, director of The Women's Nutritional Advisory Service, for the enormous amount of support she has given me over the years as a journalist writing about women's health, and whose advice and books on beating PMT through diet I heartily recommend to anyone wishing to pursue this aspect of treatment; and Dr Michael Brush, director of The Premenstrual Society, for all the encouragement, excellent advice and information he also gave me.

Introduction

'When I told my doctor I thought I was suffering with PMS, he adopted a glazed expression, then peered cynically over his specs and asked: "How old are you?"

"Forty-five!", I answered.

"Well, that's it then," he said, "you're going through the menopause." And, with that, he scribbled out a prescription for Hormone Replacement Therapy. . . .'

Jackie wasn't going through the menopause at all. But it took her over a year to get the real problem, PMS, recognized and treated. Her story is typical of women everywhere.

From virtual obscurity, PMS or PMT has become one of the most talked about twentieth-century diseases. It affects 9 out of 10 women and has over 150 symptoms. Yet, there is still an enormous amount of confusion about its causes and treatments.

I am not a doctor and I haven't made any earth-shattering scientific discoveries. I am not going to come down in favour of one theory over another about what causes PMS. Nor am I going to promote one treatment out of the many available. What I can give you in this book is the chance to learn from the experiences of the many women who kindly volunteered to talk to me about their PMS. Their stories illustrate the variety of symptoms women suffer, the range of triggers that provoke the onset of symptoms and the gamut of medical, dietary and lifestyle treatments available. Through them, I hope you will find something that helps you cope with your own PMS.

1

What is PMS?

It was 9.00 a.m. and Joyce was frantic to get to work. Not because she was afraid of being late and certainly not because she was eager to get started on her month's end accounts, but because she was gasping for a drink of hot chocolate.

Dumping her coat and bag on her desk, she charged into the office kitchen and fiddled clumsily with the sachet of chocolate powder as she waited impatiently for the kettle to boil. Seconds later, the drink was ready and Joyce's relief was instant as she took her first, long, sip.

She was still savouring the moment when the cleaning lady popped her head round the door.

'Hot chocolate, at this time of day?' she teased.

'Yes,' Joyce laughed, 'I could have murdered for it this morning!' Then she added, 'I bet you anything I'm exactly ten days off from my period.'

Joyce recalls: 'The cleaning lady looked completely baffled as I rushed back to my desk and returned with my diary. "Told you so!" I said as we both stared at my chart. There, in black and white was my period, marked with a cross, exactly ten days ahead.'

Joyce has suffered from premenstrual syndrome (PMS) for as long as she can remember. She knows her 28-day menstrual cycle off by heart, and can guarantee that the first sign of trouble is desperate chocolate craving ten days before her period is due.

'It's downhill from that day on', she says. 'I become weepy, clumsy and forgetful. My breasts balloon to three or four times their normal size – it's the only time I have a decent bust! They are also incredibly sore and painful. I have to warn my husband off coming anywhere near them. Even brushing against someone is agonizingly painful.'

Joyce is a classic sufferer of PMS. The sore and swollen breasts, chocolate cravings, weepiness and clumsiness are all typical symptoms, and Joyce knows it.

Having identified the problem, she has been able to talk to her doctor about it and now receives the treatment she needs to keep her symptoms under control. If only it were that easy for everyone.

PMS is the most common illness to affect women of childbearing age – nine out of ten women suffer it to some degree at some point in their lives. But many of us go years before recognizing the problem. How can that be?

One reason is that every woman's experience of PMS is different, and it is therefore difficult to draw comparisons or to diagnose clearly every case.

PMS has around 150 symptoms that may appear alone or in batches in the days – or, in some cases, weeks – leading up to a period. These symptoms may be mild and hardly noticeable or so severe that they seriously hamper your life, making you feel like a Jekyll and Hyde character: the person you like to think of as the 'real' you for the first half of your monthly cycle; and someone completely unrecognizable for the second half of the month.

This unrecognizable self may be irrational, moody, withdrawn, sensitive, argumentative (just a few of the psychological symptoms). She may also be bloated, spotty, greasy haired and craving chocolates and alcohol. Not the kind of person you'd invite to take over your life and meet new people on your behalf, but, for some women, there appears to be no choice in the matter – the monster takes over regardless of whether they want her to or not.

The reason so many of us have a problem identifying our PMS is that, of the 150 symptoms on the menu, we may have sampled only a few and these may not be recognizable as PMS to us until we meet or hear about someone whose experience appears to mirror our own who has identified PMS as being the problem.

To complicate matters further, although PMS is, by definition, cyclical – that is to say it always occurs in the final days of your menstrual cycle, just before your period starts – this pattern may not be obvious if your cycle is irregular, taking a different format every month.

The severity and duration of symptoms also varies enormously between women. And it is, unfortunately, the most severe forms of PMS that are often the hardest to recognize. This is because, in the worst cases, premenstrual mood swings, aggression and violence are mistaken for mental illness.

If you feel out of control and are then told by your doctor that you need to see a psychiatrist, you are unlikely to turn around and say, 'No, you're wrong, this is PMS!' – *unless someone has already shown you that it might be.*

In this book we hear some horrendous stories from women who believed they were mad/possessed/not worthy of living. They had no idea they were suffering PMS or, more importantly, that the root of their illness could be treated, until they read articles or saw TV programmes about other PMS sufferers and, finally, put two and two together. That moment, as many of them explain, was a major turning point. They had seen the light at the end of the tunnel and knew that they were finally going to be able to turn their lives around.

The point of these stories is not to frighten, but to encourage. I want to show you how versatile and complicated PMS can be. And, from the experiences of other women related on these pages, I hope to help you identify – or rule out – your own symptoms as PMS.

The history of PMS – recognizing the problem

PMS is not a new condition – it has been around as long as women have – but it has only relatively recently come out of the closet. Why is this?

One reason is that women tend to have fewer children these days than they did 100 or even 50 years ago. When women spent more of their childbearing years pregnant or nursing babies, their periods came in such short intervals of their life that any PMS symptoms they experienced were fleeting and soon forgotten with the next pregnancy.

There is also the fact that our twentieth-century diet and lifestyle appear to be making our symptoms worse. We consume far too much sugar, salt and animal fats. Also our bodies are under extra stress from the pollutants we have to cope with – lead in petrol and pesticides in crop sprays. PMS is a classic example of a twentieth-century disease (and later in this book, we will see how simple dietary and lifestyle changes can, in many cases, relieve the monthly misery of PMS).

But, even as a twentieth-century disease, PMS really seems to have come into its own in the last 15 years. A major reason for this is that menstrual problems have not been discussed openly until relatively recently.

For one thing, menstruation has never been the kind of thing women have wanted to boast about.

Hundreds of years back, if you'd lived in certain ancient tribes, you would have been locked away during your period because it was believed that, during menstruation, women developed evil powers and were at risk of casting spells on their menfolk and even killing off whole herds of animals.

Some modern religions still regard a menstruating woman as undesirable. Muslim women are not allowed to enter the mosque when they have their period. And Orthodox Jewish women are not permitted to sleep with their husbands at this time of month.

Even if you have not been raised in one of these religions, you may have been brought up to think of your periods as a 'personal time', which shouldn't be discussed.

It is only since women have become more open about their symptoms, finally recognizing that PMS is nothing to be ashamed of, that the problem has been given a good airing.

The turning point came when PMS made the headlines in 1981. That year, two women, both facing charges for serious criminal offences, pleaded in their defence that they were suffering from PMS.

Christine English was a 37-year-old divorced mother of 2 children who killed her lover after an argument, by running him over with her car.

Just before the accident he had walked away from her and stuck two fingers up at her as he left.

In a statement to the police she said that she was already mad

6

with her lover and when he gestured at her she 'just snapped', jamming her foot on the accelerator, intending to bump into him and shut him up. She certainly hadn't meant to kill him. She was suffering from PMS at the time, which she claimed gave her a diminished sense of responsibility. The court accepted that she had committed the crime under 'wholly exceptional circumstances' and Mrs English was given a conditional discharge and banned from driving for 12 months.

Sandie Smith was a 29-year-old barmaid who threatened to kill a policeman with a knife. She was already on probation for stabbing a 19-year-old girl to death the previous year. The judge told the court that she was not responsible for her actions, 'because her illness [PMS] had affected her brain'.

PMS today – the new debate

For women of my generation, growing up before the syndrome hit the news, PMS, or PMT as it used to be known, was part of 'the curse' that, as women, we were going to have to live with.

The cases that made it front-page news were a godsend. They proved there was more to a woman's premenstrual phase than a bit of tension. The new name, Premenstrual Syndrome, was adopted and PMS became a recognized complaint. Women began to talk about it, to compare notes and to identify their own symptoms.

The down-side to all this publicity has been the idea, in certain quarters, that women are now encouraged to succumb to PMS and to perform badly at work during their premenstrual phase.

The whole notion of PMS, feminists claim, has done a lot of damage to women.

It is true that some male employers think all women are below par prior to their period and are therefore reluctant to offer a woman a job that a man might do just as well and remain on an even keel throughout the month.

Sadly the debate is fuelled by some (but mercifully not all) family doctors. Many of these GPs received their training before PMS was given a decent space on the agenda, so it is still possible to see a doctor who dismisses your symptoms as 'all in the mind'.

Maryon Stewart, director of the Women's Nutritional Advisory Service, recalls a particularly chauvinistic doctor who advised a premenstrual patient to join the Conservative Party and become a Magistrate. It had apparently worked wonders for his wife. Probably because it got her away from him!

The argument against PMS is supported by Professor John Richardson, who has studied PMS for 15 years, and believes female mood swings should *not* be linked with the monthly cycle. He argues that it's not that women *don't* experience these emotional symptoms because, obviously, they do, but that there is no evidence to link them to the hormonal changes involved in the menstrual cycle.

What seems to happen, he says, is that, if a woman feels under par around her period, she – and often her partner – blame PMS. But when she feels depressed or can't concentrate at other times, she blames something else – such as her partner!

Professor Richardson believes women feel less able and more easily upset around their period because society *expects* them to feel that way. But, in fact, they aren't, and he backs up his argument by saying that he conducted a study in which pre-menstrual women were given a fake drug and 84 per cent of them reported a considerable improvement.

But does their response to the placebo drug *really* mean that their PMS was all in their mind in the first place? As many PMS sufferers discover, symptoms are less severe when they are on holiday or feeling relaxed. So, if a doctor gives you a drug and says, 'this will make you feel better', some of the pressure is instantly lifted off them and so they are quite likely to report that there has been some improvement. But, used long term, a placebo is unlikely to be so effective!

The case for PMS is, fortunately, supported by a number of specialists – among them Dr Katharina Dalton, who has been studying and treating the syndrome for over 30 years.

Dr Dalton agrees that men – and women – sometimes wrongly put women's behaviour down to PMS, but that does not mean that the syndrome merely has a psychological and social basis. Millions of women *do* have it and it's important to accept and try to understand this disorder. It's a reminder that Mother Nature still has to iron out a few flaws.

She points out that the effects of PMS are severe. Idyllic marriages can break up if a wife is regularly unpredictable, irrational and even violent. And women's work performance is affected on a day-to-day basis.

Her argument is supported by a study of 1561 boarding school girls whose weekly grades showed that the quality of schoolgirls' work dropped by 10 per cent in the week before their period. Equally significant, she adds, is the fact that the rate of attempted suicide among women is seven times higher in the second half of the menstrual cycle and shoplifting is 30 times more common at that time.

'Women who commit crimes while suffering from PMS deserve our sympathy and treatment. Of course, there will always be those who try to jump on the PMS bandwagon, but we still need to help those women imprisoned for crimes committed when they were not in control.'

You can be sure it is PMS if your symptoms start between 3 and 14 days *before* your period, and stop soon after the onset of bleeding.

Althea, Public Relations Officer for the National Association for Premenstrual Syndrome, says:

I truly thought I was mad – and I was relieved beyond belief when my PMS was diagnosed and treated and I became my old self again. So you can imagine how I feel when someone tells me PMS doesn't exist. In fact, one of our best friends recently said just that, and my husband told him straight: 'Fine, if you don't believe in PMS, I'll deliver her to your home and you can see for yourself. Live with her for a month without her medication and diet, but promise me one thing – you don't bring her back to me until she's back on her treatment.'

The advice in this book is not aimed at anyone wishing to prove her problems are *not* premenstrual. It is for the very many, like Joyce and Althea, who need to establish that their symptoms *are* due to PMS in order to get the treatment they need to free their lives of monthly misery.

Back to basics – what causes PMS?

We know far more today about the way our bodies work than our mothers or grandmothers ever did.

We know that during the first half of our menstrual cycle (which starts on the first day of a period), our bodies produce a surge of oestrogen, the upbeat, sexy and excitable female hormone. And that during the second half of the cycle (the premenstrual phase), a wave of progesterone, the downbeat, frumpy hormone, comes into play. This is fine, providing that the hormones are well balanced.

Symptoms of PMS appear at the time when we are (or should be) experiencing a rise in progesterone levels. This suggests that a hormonal imbalance – either too much oestrogen or too little progesterone – at this time is aggravating normal physical and psychological changes and turning them into unpleasant symptoms. But, we still do not know exactly what causes the hormonal imbalances behind PMS, though we do know there are various factors involved.

Is it a fault in the hypothalamus, which controls the hormonal changes that take place during the menstrual cycle?

Is it a problem in the pituitary gland, one step down the hormonal circuit from the hypothalamus, which releases leading hormones?

Are we releasing too little progesterone at the end of our cycle, when progesterone levels are supposed to be going up? Or has our oestrogen level failed to drop, or even gone up instead of down?

Are we deficient in essential fatty acids, which contribute to the production of the prolactin hormone?

Is the liver letting us down by failing to sort our wasted hormones into good and bad and leaving us with the wrong balance at the end of our cycle?

Is the normal release of the downbeat hormone progesterone

dragging up all sorts of unresolved anxieties, which we have never got around to dealing with?

These are a few of the theories behind PMS that experts have put forward and which we will explore in this book.

The way I see it, it is possible that any of these theories will be accurate, for some sufferers. But none of them is the definitive answer for everyone.

Your own PMS may have one cause or many. The point is, we are all different. Indeed, you are less likely to establish exactly what *causes* your own PMS than you are to discover exactly what *treats* it.

As each treatment – whether it be hormonal therapy, vitamin supplements, or a better diet – is based on a different theory about the cause of PMS, my advice is to be as open-minded as possible and work your way through the ones that most appeal to you (and even those that don't) until you find something that makes you feel better.

The best approach is to start with simple treatments and, only if necessary, work your way through to the more invasive treatments available.

Knowing what we do about doctors' attitudes to 'women's troubles' and having a good idea of the reception our complaint will get when we seek help, it is hardly surprising that so many of us are reluctant to acknowledge our PMS, preferring to plod on and ignore any symptoms until they become unbearable. Your symptoms may even appear to indicate that you are mentally unbalanced. But, if they are cyclical, they can probably be treated.

Joyce says:

Premenstrually I felt like a balloon slowly filling up with hot air. Not only was my tummy bloated, but I felt as if my head was about to explode. The day my bleeding started was always an enormous relief. All the hot air evaporated and I was back down to my normal size and normal state of mind.

I felt such a freak until I read about women who were crashing their cars, shoplifting and beating their husbands up before their period. I always thought I was a Jekyll and Hyde character, but other women suffered even *more* than me . . . I felt sorry for them, but relieved by the sense that there's security in numbers. If they'd suffered so badly and still managed to overcome their symptoms I had absolutely no excuse for sitting on my backside and doing nothing about my own PMS. In fact, I owed it to women everywhere to make sure I got the treatment I needed. Because, the more women insisted on treatment for, and recognition of PMS, the more doctors would have to start taking us seriously.

2

How can you be sure it's PMS?

Recognizing the symptoms

The following remarks were made by five different women who suffer from PMS.

I am so clumsy – one minute I'm holding a glass, the next minute it's on the floor. And I haven't a clue why I dropped it!

I'm completely absent-minded: I put my house keys in my car door, and my bus pass in the autobank machine. I've even shown my train ticket to the security guard at the office. I don't seem to be able to keep my mind on anything!

I'm a driving instructor, but premenstrually I have so little confidence in my driving I will sit for ten minutes at a junction, not knowing when to move out!

I feel so insecure before my period that an acquaintance only has to respond distractedly for me to feel that the whole world is against me.

I'm like a raging bull when my period's due – and woe betide anyone who steps in my way!

All five women suffer emotional and/or psychological symptoms of PMS, but each has a different experience premenstrually.

The following are descriptions of typical physical symptoms.

I can't stand the thought of sex for about five days before my period.

My breasts are so sore that nothing I wear feels comfortable.

My stomach gets so big, that I have to wear clothes with elasticated waistbands.

13

For a week before my period, I am constantly hungry. My husband can't stand it. He calls it pigishness.

I know my period is due when I develop mouth ulcers. Eating is uncomfortable for about four days, then, as soon as my bleeding starts, the ulcers vanish!

What a shame that there is no *single* symptom that is characteristic of *all* cases of PMS! It would make it so much easier for sufferers and their doctors to identify the problem.

But, if any of the above comments ring a bell with you and if you can prove that the symptoms you recognize *only* occur premenstrually, you are probably one of the 90 per cent of women who suffer PMS.

Over 150 symptoms of PMS are recognized by experts, but the most common are:

- feeling depressed, sad, or pessimistic
- feeling under par, tired or lethargic
- tension, irritability and anxiety
- a change in appetite
- cravings for sugary or salty foods
- feeling thirstier than usual
- lacking in concentration
- indecisiveness
- weepiness
- mood swings
- feeling extra sexy or losing interest in sex
- sleeping badly
- aggression
- impulsiveness
- increased energy
- loss of confidence and self-esteem
- feelings of guilt
- feelings that you are inadequate
- loss of interest in yourself
- feeling that you can't be bothered with anything
- headaches and migraine

- swollen, tender breasts
- bloating
- swollen fingers and toes
- acne, rashes and itching
- constipation, nausea or diarrhoea
- clumsiness
- muscle weakness and backache
- dizziness
- weight gain
- sweatiness
- sore eyes
- a change in the amount of urine you pass
- abdominal cramps
- increased vaginal discharge
- feeling less efficient than usual.

Professor Guy Abrahams, formerly Professor of Obstetrics and Gynaecology at the University of California and now Patron of the Women's Nutritional Advisory Service, has identified four types of PMS sufferer:

- type A experiencing anxiety, irritability, tension

- type B experiencing bloating, swelling, weight gain

- type C experiencing cravings for sweets and stodgy foods followed by exhaustion, headache, and fainting brought on by sudden rises and falls in blood sugar (hypoglycaemia).

- type D experiencing depression and confusion.

Most sufferers experience symptoms from more than one of these groups.

Nervous tension, anxiety, irritability and mood swings are thought to be caused by elevated levels of oestrogen in the premenstrual phase, due to a vitamin B_6 deficiency. The liver,

15

which breaks down the body's waste products, needs healthy supplies of vitamin B_6 in order to get rid of the portion of oestrogen that is no longer needed in the second half of the menstrual cycle. If, for some reason, you are lacking the necessary levels of vitamin B_6, the liver cannot do its job properly and oestrogen builds up in the body.

Too much oestrogen is thought to cause an imbalance in brain chemicals and overproduction of stimulating chemicals, such as serotonin, adrenaline and noradrenaline, and underproduction of the soothing chemicals, such as dopamine.

When these chemicals are out of balance, you are likely to feel irritable and uptight and to suffer dramatic mood swings. These mood swings mean that, between being bad-tempered and aggressive, you may be drowsy and incapable of performing everyday tasks at your normal capacity.

Bloating, swelling and weight gain are caused by fluid retention, which is also a symptom of too much oestrogen. Even dieters may notice that their weight, which has been steadily falling, suddenly increases premenstrually.

Scientists have worked out that oestrogen causes the body to retain high levels of sodium, which is found in salt. The sodium causes water to remain in the body and, instead of being excreted in the usual way, it finds its way into other parts of the body – causing fingers to swell, breasts to balloon, waistlines to expand and ankles to thicken up.

Swelling in the nose can make you feel stuffy, as if you have a cold. And a build-up of water in the sinuses may produce a vacuum headache.

Cravings and attacks of nausea and tiredness are a common feature of PMS and are symptoms of hypoglycaemia – low blood sugar level – attacks. The question is, why should premenstrual women experience hypoglycaemic attacks more than anyone else?

What normally happens is that our blood sugar level rises quickly after eating and then falls gradually over a period of hours until the next meal, by which time our blood sugar level has reached its 'baseline' and we are usually feeling tired and in need of pepping up. (You only have to look at the way a grumpy child comes back to life after a sandwich and a drink at teatime, to see the immediate effects food has on our blood sugar level.)

Premenstrually, it seems that changes in the hormone levels affect our normal sugar tolerance, causing the blood sugar baseline to rise so that we cannot manage to go as long as we normally would without food. One way of getting the quick burst of energy your body is telling you it needs is to eat something sweet. Hence, a lot of women experience chocolate cravings at this time in the month. Unfortunately, however, chocolate and sugary foods actually exacerbate the problem. They give you short bursts of excitable high energy, followed by a sudden fit of weakness, lethargy and hunger (as the blood sugar level drops suddenly back), which make you crave even *more* chocolate or sugar. Soon you are locked into a vicious circle of cravings and attacks of nausea.

How can you get round this problem? See the dietary advice in Chapter 6.

Depression and confusion, insomnia and weepiness are caused not by the *high* levels of oestrogen linked to other symptoms of PMS, but by *low* levels during the first half of the menstrual cycle. One reason for these low levels is thought to be that lead poisoning, which has been linked to depression, blocks the production of oestrogen. Stress is also thought to affect the production of this hormone and, indeed, many PMS sufferers report that their symptoms are aggravated when they are under stress.

Symptoms of PMS may be mild and hardly noticeable, as in Kerry's experience.

I don't keep tabs on my menstrual cycle, which means I never have any idea when my period is due. But on a number of occasions I have convinced myself I am pregnant because all my symptoms seem to point to pregnancy. My breasts are fuller, but not at all painful. I feel mildly nauseous when I wake up and I have to go to the loo more frequently than usual.

Around the same time I may become short-tempered and very sensitive to criticism – but I don't see this as in any way out of character until my period arrives, and, looking back, suddenly I can't see what all the fuss was about. I also recognize, but only retrospectively, that I didn't have symptoms of pregnancy but of PMS.

They may be moderate, as Helen has found.

I was first aware of my PMS when I was at university. It was my friends who spotted it. People used to say, 'You're very cranky today!' I remembered my mother saying the same thing. She used to tell me I was 'impossible' – and I soon came to realize that I was always impossible and cranky on the day before my period.

As I've got older I've realized my PMS is much worse when I'm tired or under strain. If I'm on holiday I can sail through it with no trouble.

The first sign is a gripey tummyache about a week before my period is due. That's always a pretty bad warning – and I know that I'm going to get steadily worse over the next seven days.

As my period approaches, I have to try not to do anything that involves too much thought. I get calculations wrong and make silly mistakes that I would never normally let pass.

The day before my period is the worst. I am very irritable and get angry at the slightest thing. I am completely critical of everyone and everything and burst into tears very easily.

My poor husband can't do a thing right. I see him trying to tread carefully to keep out of my way and not do anything that will set me off – and that only gets me more upset. I must be impossible to live with.

Just before my period, I have terrible difficulty getting off to sleep, and I wake up feeling tired and unsatisfied. But, on the first day of bleeding, I sleep really well and feel instantly better.

Your symptoms may be very severe, as in Althea's case.

As far as I can recall, my PMS started when I was going through a rough time in my life. My father had recently died, my husband had gone back to college, so we were struggling to live on his student's grant, I was working round the clock to make ends meet and we had three children all going through bad patches at school. My life was hectic and extremely stressful and I put all my own depression, constant tiredness and anxiety down to the other things going on in my life.

But, one by one, the other problems were solved. My husband was back at work, the kids were all recovering from their individual traumas and enough time had passed for me to come to terms with the loss of my father. But I was still feeling dowdy, depressed and downright boring.

When my fortieth birthday arrived with a flood of birthday cards all saying helpful things like, 'Congratulations! You're over the hill!', I thought, they're absolutely right. I *am* over the hill.

I felt old and wasted and uninteresting. I was scared of going to parties because I thought nobody would want to talk to me – my self-esteem was at rock bottom – and I suffered panic attacks. But I never put any of these symptoms down to PMS.

On one occasion, I suffered such a terrible and frightening panic attack in the middle of Hastings that my poor husband had to march me round to the casualty department of Hastings hospital and explain to an exhausted doctor that I needed help because I was refusing to get in the car.

The doctor didn't realize I was suffering from PMS – and who can blame her. She knew nothing of my history, and I hadn't put two and two together so I was in no position to help her out. So she said, 'Your wife is neurotic. Take her home and give her a very large sedative!' Eventually my husband got me home – and the next day my period started.

But, I didn't make the connection until, after going month after month to my GP about different *physical* symptoms – swollen ankles, sore boobs, chocolate cravings, acne – my doctor said, 'Do you realize you come here every month with a different symptom?! I think you've got PMS – and I think you need a progesterone treatment.'

I haven't looked back since. But when other women say, 'I feel so silly – why didn't I realize earlier that it was PMS?' I can sympathize with them completely. How are you to know that you have PMS unless someone points it out to you?'

Whether your symptoms are mild, moderate or severe, they will begin at some time between ovulation and menstruation and will last for anything from one or two days to two weeks. In some cases, they spread gradually into postmenstrual days so that there may be only one week or so left in which there are no symptoms. They may start soon after your first period or much later in life. They tend to increase in severity with age and may occur after a hysterectomy, with or without removal of the ovaries, or after sterilization or ovarian surgery.

They may also be triggered by severe illness or major physical, emotional or sexual trauma. They may occur some months and not others and they may be more severe some months than others.

In some cases, the symptoms of PMS are *so* severe that they take over the sufferer's whole life – and are not recognized as being premenstrual. Here is Carole's story.

Mood swings were ruining my life.

I always thought mood swings involved highs and lows . . . ecstasy one day, misery the next. But when my mood swings started, six years ago, the highs were few and far between.

One week out of four I felt OK. Not great, just OK. The rest of the time, I could be chugging along fairly normally – and suddenly burst into tears over what amounted to nothing. With no warning, I just snapped. I was convinced I was going mad.

I reached crisis point one fine morning when I was hanging out the washing. All that happened was I dropped a sock. But I burst into tears on the spot. If I could, I would have run away . . . but I had nowhere to run to.

In the end, I decided that what I needed more than anything else was a bit of independence. Since I had married, I'd been at home with my two young sons, Matthew and Nicholas. Now that they were going to school, I thought, a part-time job would solve all my problems.

But I didn't get a job – and nothing changed. So, in the end, I decided that there was only one thing for it. I would have to go to my doctor.

It's a terrible thing to think that you are going mad. And it is even worse to have to come out and admit it to your doctor. But I took a deep breath and explained that I kept bursting into tears, and that I felt completely and utterly sorry for myself.

I had left it so long that, by this time, there was really no relief from my mood swings. I no longer had even one good week a month when I wouldn't fly off the handle or wake up thinking I couldn't face the day.

My doctor was sympathetic, but there was little he could do except prescribe me antidepressants. I have to say, I wasn't keen on the idea. Like everyone, I had heard horror stories of women who become hooked on tranquillizers – I didn't realize antidepressants are a different kettle of fish altogether – so I was wary, but I took them anyway.

I had agreed to take the pills for a three-month trial period and when my 12 weeks were up, I was determined to get back to normal. I stopped taking them and I felt great, for a couple of days. Then, all that ghastly irritability and irrational moodiness came tumbling back. I didn't know what to do. If I really *was* mad, the only choice left to me was to see a psychiatrist.

The psychiatrist asked my about my sex life, and my marriage. And, as I answered his questions, it dawned on me that he was not going to help me at all. These areas of my life were fine. Obviously sex hadn't been that great while I had been so depressed. But I knew that it was not the cause of my bad moods.

Unhelped, I renewed my prescription for antidepressants

and stuck with them – like a washed out zombie – for the next year. Nick was incredible. Totally supportive all the way. I honestly think that anyone else would have packed their bags and gone. I was such a wet blanket.

I even began to wonder if I had ME. I'd read about it, and the symptoms sounded much like mine. All I did was mope about the house. And I woke up in the morning, just longing for the day to end so I could go back to bed again.

The children were at the age of helping in the kitchen and they liked me to make cakes with them. I tried my hardest, but I knew I was just going through the motions. Whatever I did, there was no natural enthusiasm.

But, if it hadn't been for the boys, I think I would have been suicidal. I really began to think that if this was life, then what was the point of living it? Only the thought of Matthew and Nicholas stopped me from doing something silly.

The turning point came when we decided to move house. Our new home was my dream house at that time, and it seemed like the perfect opportunity to start afresh.

I had a few antidepressant pills left and I said to Nick, 'I'm chucking these away. I won't be needing them again.' He was obviously concerned – 'Are you sure you're doing the right thing?', he asked. I knew I was. It had struck me that the only person who could help me was myself.

I booked myself some sessions with a counsellor, and she helped a bit. But what really changed my life was an article I found in a magazine. It was a woman describing her period mood swings – just like I'm doing now!

I read it, and reread it. I just couldn't believe it. This woman was describing exactly what I had been going through. It was as if she was talking about me!

Now let us hear Nicky's story.

It all started at the age of 14 when I suddenly burst into tears on my way to school one morning. I felt awful – almost suicidally depressed and very sick.

22

My mother took me to the doctor who started me, one course after the other, on antidepressants, tranquillizers, sleeping tablets, and antisickness pills. She even sent me to various child psychiatrists who all maintained that something terrible must have happened to me at the age of 14.

The only thing I could think of was that I had started my periods then. But, because I had no idea about PMS, I didn't put two and two together. And, sadly, nor did any of the doctors I saw.

My periods were always long, heavy and very irregular, so it was difficult to identify a particular pattern to my illness, but it seemed to me that I was more often ill than not.

As well as feeling extremely depressed, and so sick that I couldn't face food, or even listen to people talking about it, I suffered blinding headaches; sudden, inexplicable cravings for alcohol, chocolates and sweets (for about six months in my early thirties, I became an alcoholic because of the intensity of my cravings); hot flushes and sweating attacks; panic attacks and breathlessness; and very painful ovulation cramps, accompanied by a horrible, thick, black, mid-cycle loss of blood.

As a teenager I scoured my biology books for clues to what was wrong with me. Perhaps, with all those sugar cravings, I was diabetic? Or maybe I was epileptic? I knew that if I could only identify the illness and get the correct treatment, everything would be OK.

It wasn't until I was 29 and married with a baby daughter, that I realized what was really wrong with me. I'd suffered so badly with postnatal depression (yes, that is also linked to PMS!) that I'd been admitted for two weeks to a psychiatric hospital, and I was on a weekend break at home from the hospital when I saw a television programme about PMS.

The programme showed people suffering symptoms of acute depression – just like me. I lost my temper with everyone and would go through the house slamming every door and kicking walls.

Friends of PMS – related symptoms

The following conditions are all related, directly or indirectly, to PMS. They may be so severe in themselves that they are the problem you 'present with' when you seek help or they may be part and parcel of the complex collection of symptoms of PMS.

Loss of sex drive

Here is Debbie's story.

My husband John and I had always enjoyed sex and I felt absolutely awful when, four and a half years ago, I suddenly lost all interest in it. I had become very moody and depressed and was irritated by any approaches John made. I didn't like him touching me and kissing and cuddling were definitely out of the question.

He used to creep up behind me and kiss the back of my neck when I was cooking or washing up and I'd always enjoyed that. But, now, if I thought he was approaching, I'd quickly move out of the way. If he put his arm around me I'd shrug it off. And, in bed, I'd curl up and go to sleep before he could make a move.

When I first started to push him away, he'd look hurt and ask, 'Have I done something to upset you?' I explained that it was nothing like that, I was just tired, busy . . . any old excuse, because I couldn't face telling him the truth: I'd gone off him. It was absolutely horrible because he was still the man I loved and wanted to be with and I felt as if I was betraying him by not wanting to make love with him any more.

I was off sex for at least three months – though once or twice I thought I'd go through with it for his sake, which was always a disaster. I'd be unresponsive and he'd end up feeling even more hurt than if we'd kept up the act that I was too tired.

Eventually, of course, we were forced to a crisis point, and I had to confess how I was feeling.

Instead of thinking this was a temporary blip, John reacted badly and said, 'Oh? Do you want us to separate then?' I explained that it was just the sex, not him, and I hoped things would get back to normal in due course. But he warned me that, when I was ready for sex, I'd have to make the first move because he couldn't bear to be rejected again.

It was just by chance that, a couple of weeks after my big confession, I read about a lot of different symptoms – among them loss of sex drive, sore throats and moodiness (all things I'd suffered) – that were linked with PMS and had been solved by a change in diet.

It sounded bizarre, but, by this stage, I thought anything was worth a try.

I contacted The Women's Nutritional Advisory Service and was advised to give up smoking, caffeine, sugar and salt. I didn't think I'd manage without tea and cigarettes, but, with determination, I succeeded in giving up these 'vital' lifelines.

It took a few weeks for my symptoms to lift, but then they improved. My moodiness vanished, and one afternoon I suddenly realized that I wanted sex again.

My first thought was 'How do I break it to John?' After a few months without sex I was scared I'd be rejected if I asked him. So, I'm afraid I resorted to the corny old candle-lit supper and, over a bottle of wine, I hinted that I was 'in the mood'. At the end of the evening I said to John, 'I think I'll go to bed now', and, with a twinkle in his eye, he said, 'I think I'll join you'!

A change in sex drive is a common feature of PMS, although there are many other causes of a complete loss of interest. Some women find that their sexual energy is concentrated in the premenstrual phase of their cycle. Others, like Debbie, find it so remarkably lacking that, especially when combined with depression, it can spill over to the whole month, resulting in a total loss of libido.

For some women, the surge of progesterone in the second half of the cycle seems to diminish their sexiness, while the imput of oestrogen, after their period has come, makes them more sexual than at any other time in the month.

The body changes that occur premenstrually can also affect your sexuality. Breast tenderness can be so severe, any touching is painful. And bloating can make us feel uncomfortable and also unattractive.

As well as taking steps to rectify the hormonal imbalance and bodily changes that get in the way of a healthy sex life, you can use an experience such as premenstrual loss of libido to your advantage and make more of your natural sexual cycle (see Chapter 8 for more on this subject).

Heavy periods

Here is Tess's story.

> I never used to understand why some women called menstruation 'the curse', but then I was one of the lucky ones who had periods as regular as clockwork. They were also completely trouble-free: no cramps, and very light bleeding.
>
> Even after my daughter, Ashley, was born, in 1986, my periods went right back to how they'd been before.
>
> But then, after my son, Alexander, was born, in 1989, my periods gradually became heavier. And over 18 months or so they became so bad that for the first two days of each period, I felt as if I was haemorrhaging. I tried to be rational about it, but it was difficult not to be frightened and upset by the colossal amounts of blood I was losing.
>
> Although the first couple of days were definitely the worst each month, the blood loss remained heavy and clotted for the entire duration of the period, which usually stretched to about seven days.
>
> I hardly left the house because I was in so much discomfort. I had to wear a super tampon with a thick night-time sanitary towel. And the blood loss was so flood-like that I had to change every couple of hours because the towel was drenched.
>
> On one occasion, I remember trying to drive into town to do some shopping. I'd changed my sanitary protection before leaving the house, but, half an hour later, as I got out of my car, I could feel blood seeping through my trousers.

Fortunately, I was wearing a long tee shirt, which covered up the mark, and I rushed to the nearest loo, changed again, and drove straight back home without doing any of my shopping.

Eventually, feeling imprisoned by my heavy periods, I decided to see my GP.

As well as suffering heavy periods, I was feeling generally depressed and below par. I'd started bingeing on chocolate and I was tired and listless. Having already ruled out a medical cause, my GP said that I was obviously under stress, which could have triggered my heavy periods, and that I could stem the flow by going back on the Pill.

Reluctantly I agreed, but I wasn't at all keen on the idea. I'd already been on the Pill long enough before having my children. And, at 37, I didn't want to go back on it. My husband had even had a vasectomy, so there was really no reason, apart from my heavy periods, to start taking it again.

Miraculously, as the doctor predicted, the Pill did the trick and my periods lightened up immediately. But there was a major drawback: the listlessness, bingeing and depression all got a lot worse.

After a couple of months, I stopped taking the Pill and was back to square one, having to waddle around in heavy-duty sanitary wear, and hating every minute of it.

The turning point came when I read a magazine article about a woman who had suffered PMS. She had heavy periods, depression, chocolate cravings – all the problems that had been worrying me – and she'd treated herself by changing her diet!

It is difficult to define what is a heavy period as one woman's monthly blood loss will vary a lot throughout her life, but Tess was sufficiently worried and also hindered by her monthly periods to justify seeking medical help.

There are a number of causes of heavy periods, so you should always discuss the problem with your doctor so anything serious can be ruled out before you set about trying to treat it yourself.

The link between heavy periods and PMS is that one cause of

heavy bleeding is a hormonal imbalance, which, in Tess's case, seemed also to be producing premenstrual symptoms.

Painful ovulation

Here is Angela's story.

Some women are so in tune with their monthly cycles that they know exactly when they should be ovulating (releasing an egg). And it probably comes as no surprise to them if the process is painful. But, when I first began to experience these low abdominal pains – about five years ago – I had no idea what was wrong with me.

My periods had always been a problem. Right from the beginning – when I was 14 – they were too far apart. I would go up to 48 days without bleeding. And then, when my period came, it would be extremely heavy. For the first few days I would be literally flooded with blood!

The problem was, as my periods were irregular, I never knew when to expect one. So, the first couple of times I experienced painful ovulation, I believed it was just the onset of my period. The pain was very similar to a period pain. It would start as a small ache in my groin and build up to a feeling of strangulation, as if my abdomen was being squeezed very tightly. This would drag on for up to five days. It would have been easy to give in to it and put myself to bed, but I'm a bit of a trouper and tend to carry on as best I can. Especially as I thought I was waiting for my period to start, going to bed seemed a little dramatic! But, all this time, nothing would happen, and my period would eventually come another ten days later.

When this became a regular (or as regular as could be expected with my irregular cycle) occurrence, I began to worry. I started to think that the pain was nothing to do with my menstrual cycle, and that, instead, I must have cancer.

As time was going on, the cramps were becoming more severe, and I took this as a sign that something was definitely wrong.

I had never had anyone to talk to me about these kinds of problems. I was 34, but had grown up quite ignorant about my own body. My mother was not the type to talk about periods – and, even if she had suffered with them, she didn't tell me about it. So, the whole experience was completely new to me.

With the increasing severity of the pains, I found myself becoming paranoid. I was convinced I was going to die. What I didn't realize at the time was that I was suffering from chronic premenstrual syndrome. The painful ovulation seemed to be the trigger point. For the ten days between these midcycle pains and my period, I was in complete turmoil – convinced I was either going mad or I had genuinely little time to live.

My GP was understanding and said that, although I had a long and stretched out menstrual cycle, the pains I was suffering were probably due to ovulation. He also suggested that PMS was adding to my problems during the second half of my cycle.

When he said this, I could see the pattern emerging. But before that I had no idea why sometimes I was my old bubbly, outgoing self, while the rest of the time I felt a complete weed!

The doctor would normally have treated the problem with the Pill, but, because of a heart complaint, I can't use the Pill. So he offered me a hysterectomy instead.

As far as I was concerned, a hysterectomy was not a life-saving operation and I decided to try other things before taking such drastic action.

In fact, I changed my diet and lifestyle and, in so doing, have managed to get rid of my mid-month pains. My periods are much lighter too, although they are still pretty haphazard.

Ovulation is the natural process that takes place in any fertile woman whose body is going through its normal cycle of preparing for pregnancy. It is the development and release of an ovum (egg) from a follicle within the ovary, which occurs during the middle of the menstrual cycle, on about the 11th or 14th day.

Signs of ovulation include a rise in body temperature and changes in the amount and consistency of cervical mucus. Painful ovulation (the correct name is Mittelschmerz) is not usually severe. In most women who suffer at all (and many do not) the pain is on one side of the abdomen and lasts only a few hours. Slight spotting (vaginal blood loss) may accompany the pain.

At its most severe, Mittelschmerz can feel like a needle-piercing pain, combined with cramp, that can last for several days – as in Angela's case.

Painful ovulation is not part of PMS; it is a separate issue. Some women have PMS without painful ovulation. Others have never had PMS, but know every month, because of the pain, that they are ovulating. However, if you suffer both, you are probably more aware than others of your painful ovulation because, when it comes, it heralds that the horrors of PMS are ahead. In some women who suffer from severely painful ovulation, this can last for a week. They then have a week of PMS and a week of (often painful) periods. That leaves them with only one week of relative 'normality', so they are, not surprisingly, acutely aware of the different problems that plague their cycle.

'Is it PMS?'

Identifying your PMS may be the first step in solving a lot of your problems. If you suffer from any of the symptoms described in this chapter, you could have PMS. But, remember, these symptoms may also have *other* causes and treating your PMS may not solve everything. Other factors in your life – stress, exhaustion, overwork, marital difficulties, problems with your children and so on – may all be entirely genuine and treating your PMS will not always magic *all* of them better. But, if PMS is making your situation any worse than it should be, you will be doing yourself a tremendous favour if you can identify it, treat it and take it out of the equation.

PMS can make you forgetful and irrational. Remove it and you will at least be in a position to make informed decisions, on an even keel, about any other areas of your life that may need tackling.

3

Understanding the causes

Why do some women get PMS while others do not?

Sarah has suffered PMS, in varying degrees of intensity, for most of her adult life. Her symptoms – bloated stomach, sore breasts and horrendous mood swings – mean she knows exactly when her period is due. And she is tremendously relieved when it eventually comes.

Sarah's sister, Jane, on the other hand, has never experienced PMS.

Both women are married with children. Both have stressful jobs and both have their fair share of money worries. They are the same weight (except premenstrually, when Sarah piles on the pounds) and the same height.

So why is it that Sarah suffers and Jane doesn't?

The fact is, nobody really knows.

Not only are doctors still divided about whether or not PMS exists in the first place, but there is also major confusion among doctors who do believe in PMS about what causes some women and not others to suffer.

The most obvious reason seems to be individual variation. Just as, within a family, one person can be taller or shorter than their brothers and sisters, and another can be the odd one out, having freckles or hairy legs, say, our internal systems can work differently from those of our sisters, mothers and grandmothers, too.

It seems that some of us are simply more vulnerable than others to the many factors – diet, lifestyle, pollution – that seem to play some part in blocking or increasing the production of key hormones.

Even if *all* the female members of *one* family suffer PMS, each of their symptoms may stem from a different cause or originate in

31

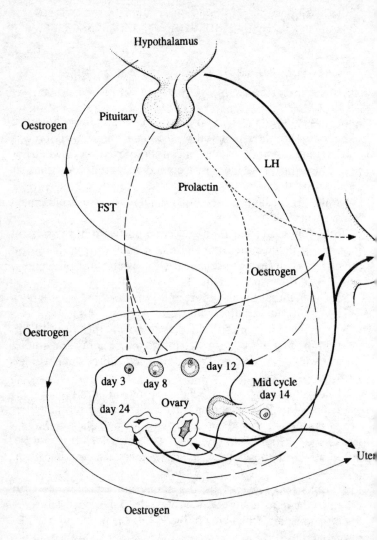

a different point in the menstrual cycle. And it is because there are so many possible causes of PMS that finding the most suitable treatment can sometimes be a long and drawn out process.

Understanding your menstrual cycle

Although the exact causes of PMS have not been identified, we do know that it is linked to the hormonal changes that take place during the menstrual cycle.

In a normal, healthy and fertile woman, the menstrual cycle usually lasts around 28 days (although slightly shorter or longer cycles are still acceptable and entirely normal).

The cycle follows the same pattern every month (unless pregnancy takes place), developing and releasing an ovum (egg) from a follicle within the ovary. The release of the ovum is called ovulation and takes place during the middle of the menstrual cycle – usually between days 10 and 14 of a typical 28-day cycle.

As the egg grows each month, it develops inside a small cyst, or follicle. By the time it is ready to be released, this cyst will have grown to about 2.5 cm (1 in) in diameter. If you are examined on an ultrasound scan immediately prior to ovulation, the cyst would show up as being on the ovary. This is entirely normal.

When the cyst ruptures, the fluid from it leaks into the abdominal cavity. There can also be some blood escaping with the fluid from the cyst and this, too, will normally spill into the abdomen and remain internally, to be disposed of through the body's natural waste systems.

The egg then begins its journey through the Fallopian tubes, to the uterus.

If it is not fertilized, the egg dies and is disposed of with its accompanying blood and mucous in the next period, at which point the cycle starts all over again.

The role of hormones in the cycle

Throughout the monthly cycle, there is an enormous amount of hormonal activity and your body undergoes an amazing number of changes.

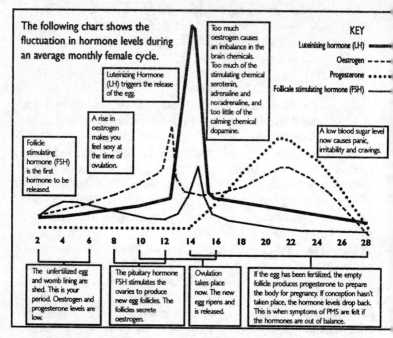

The following chart shows the fluctuation in hormone levels during an average monthly female cycle.

KEY
Luteinising hormone (LH) ▬▬▬
Oestrogen ▬ ▬ ▬
Progesterone • • • • •
Follicle stimulating hormone (FSH) ▬▬▬

Luteinizing Hormone (LH) triggers the release of the egg.

Too much oestrogen causes an imbalance in the brain chemicals. Too much of the stimulating chemical serotenin, adrenaline and noradrenaline, and too little of the calming chemical dopamine.

A rise in oestrogen makes you feel sexy at the time of ovulation.

Follicle stimulating hormone (FSH) is the first hormone to be released.

A low blood sugar level now causes panic, irritability and cravings.

The unfertilized egg and womb lining are shed. This is your period. Oestrogen and progesterone levels are low.

The pituitary hormone FSH stimulates the ovaries to produce new egg follicles. The follicles secrete oestrogen.

Ovulation takes place now. The new egg ripens and is released.

If the egg has been fertilized, the empty follicle produces progesterone to prepare the body for pregnancy. If conception hasn't taken place, the hormone levels drop back. This is when symptoms of PMS are felt if the hormones are out of balance.

    The coordination of these changes is timed with the precision of a busy airport runway. The control centre is the hypothalamus, a small cherry-shaped structure in the brain, responsible for sending chemical messengers (hormones) all over the body. The hypothalamus is connected to the pituitary gland by a short stalk of nerve fibres and controls the secretion of hormones from the pituitary.

    It kicks off the menstrual cycle by sending a message to the pituitary gland, giving it the go-ahead to produce its own hormones. The first of these is known as follicle stimulating hormone (FSH), which is carried in the bloodstream to the ovaries. Once there, as its name implies, it stimulates the growth of the follicle within which the egg develops.

    As the egg grows, the walls of the follicle produce increasing amounts of the female hormone, oestrogen. This starts to build up the lining of the uterus (womb) and causes a rise in sexual interest as the level of oestrogen in the blood builds up to a peak just before ovulation.

The pituitary now releases another hormone, luteinizing hormone (LH), that triggers the release of the mature egg (ovulation). As the egg begins to travel from the ovary through the Fallopian tubes to the uterus, the LH causes the follicle to become a solid yellow mass (corpus luteum), which produces large amounts of the hormone progesterone, the main function of which is to prepare the lining of the uterus to receive the fertilized egg.

If the egg is not fertilized, the pituitary, responding to the high level of oestrogen and progesterone produced by the corpus luteum in the ovary, now lowers its production of LH. This drop in LH causes the corpus luteum to decay, and the levels of progesterone and oestrogen then fall, too.

What is happening to the cycle when PMS occurs?

The symptoms of PMS take place when, during the latter half of the cycle – after ovulation has taken place – there is either too much or too little of certain hormones.

Theories about PMS

Too little progesterone

One of the most popular theories about PMS is that it is due to a deficiency of the hormone progesterone in relation to the amount of oestrogen in the body in the second half of the cycle.

A lot of women benefit greatly from treatment with progesterone therapy, which boosts supplies of progesterone at this crucial stage in the cycle. However this treatment does not work for everyone, and some women with very severe symptoms of PMS have perfectly normal levels of progesterone.

Too much oestrogen

Excessively high levels of oestrogen (in relation to progesterone) are thought to be capable of causing depression and mood swings. Oestrogen interferes with the body's absorption of vitamin B_6, which is known as the antidepression vitamin because it controls the production of a compound called serotonin. Serotonin is essential for brain and nerve function and an inadequate supply causes depression.

Too much prolactin

Prolactin is the hormone produced by the pituitary gland to regulate levels of oestrogen and progesterone. It also stimulates the breasts to produce milk when you have had a baby. Too much prolactin can make your breasts sore and enlarged and upset the delicate balance of progesterone and oestrogen.

Too few essential fatty acids

Studies have shown that where essential fatty acids (EFAs) are in short supply, the body is abnormally sensitive to small changes in hormonal levels, producing the same symptoms you would get if you have an excess of prolactin.

Too little vitamin B_6

We have already seen that a hormone imbalance can affect the way your body uses its supplies of vitamin B_6. Vitamin B_6, in turn, increases the efficiency with which your body makes use of EFAs. If you have a hormone imbalance, you may need more than the usual amount of vitamin B_6 in your diet.

A problem with the hypothalamus

Imagine the hormones are the planes taking off and landing at our busy airport, and that each of these is in perfect working order, with an A1 pilot in the cockpit. If a crash still occurs, you would probably start your investigation back in the air traffic control centre.

Like the air traffic control centre, the hypothalamus is responsible for receiving messages and sending new ones out. It only has to get one or two lines crossed during the menstrual cycle and your normal hormonal activity will be sent off course, causing PMS.

The hypothalamus is involved with numerous hormonal changes around the body, from controlling blood sugar levels to stimulating growth of bone and muscle tissue and starting off the contractions we experience during labour.

It also stimulates parts of the nervous system, affecting:

- heart rate
- blood pressure
- heat regulation (sweating, shivering)
- muscular movement in the stomach and intestines
- constriction and relaxation of the bronchial tubes in the lungs.

The hypothalamus also regulates eating habits by registering hunger and satisfaction. It controls body-weight and holds the key to emotions such as rage, anxiety and fear.

If you compare the areas where the hypothalamus is involved with the list of PMS symptoms given on page 14, it seems quite likely that, in many sufferers, the cause lies in a faulty hypothalamus. Unfortunately, nobody knows, yet, why the hypothalamus may start to play up, but we do know that the hypothalamus operates by means of feedback – that is, by responding to what is already happening in the body. So:

- if your body temperature is too high or too low, it will introduce sweating or shivering to bring it back within the normal range
- it responds to neurotransmitters, the substances we secrete under stress and that are related to mood changes, which shows how stress and mood can bring about hormonal changes
- it is also affected by trauma, nutrition and infection
- deficiencies in progesterone, prostaglandin, vitamins, magnesium and endorphins are all related to changes in the activity of the hypothalamus
- so are excesses of oestrogen and prolactin
- low blood sugar level (which occurs when you go a long time

without food), fluid retention and stress are also likely to affect the hypothalamus.

A problem with the pituitary

One step further down the line, it is possible that an underactive pituitary gland is at the root of some women's PMS. A poor diet can cause the pituitary to decrease activity and, in severe cases, periods may stop altogether. Physical or emotional stress can also cause the pituitary to put its feet up and stop working as hard as it should.

Finding the triggers

By charting your symptoms on a day-by-day monthly chart over the course of three months, you will be able to identify a pattern to your PMS. You may realize, for example, that you are always sensitive to remarks other people make four days before your period, argumentative and explosive two days before onset of bleeding and fluey on the day before it starts.

Once you have identified the pattern, it is usually possible to trace back to the time of its onset. This may have been a time when you were undergoing hormonal change – the start of your periods, the birth of one of your children or the introduction of new hormones via use of the Pill. It may be related to a particularly stressful life event – the death of a loved one, the end of a relationship, the loss of your home or job. Or it could be linked to an overall change in your lifestyle – a different diet or a striking increase or reduction in the amount of exercise you take. Often, it is not until something happens to return things to the way they were before you ever suffered PMS that you are able to make the connection.

Factors that can predispose you to PMS by causing problems with your fluctuating hormone levels include:

- stressful life events (such as illness, marital discord, overwork and so on)

- childbirth, though not necessarily after the first baby
- postnatal depression
- recent gynaecological operations or a miscarriage or abortion
- drinking alcohol and smoking cigarettes
- pollution (because coping with it drains your natural supply of PMS-fighting nutrients)
- gynaecological disorders (such as endometriosis or ovarian cysts)
- underlying psychiatric disorders (such as a family history of mental illness)
- lack of exercise
- a diet of processed (especially sugary) foods
- long-term use of the Pill can sometimes cause small deficiencies in your nutritional stocks, which can build up unnoticed because the Pill stops ovulation, but which will give you sudden PMS when you finally come off the Pill
- your age (PMS symptoms are known to get worse as the years go by)
- allergy to certain foods.

Let us look at some examples of these factors.

Fiona's story shows how PMS can start as early as at the onset of puberty.

I have suffered from PMS for as long as I have been having periods. But my behaviour was so bizarre that doctors thought I was mentally unbalanced and I, being none the wiser, went along with what they said.

Then, four years ago, I became pregnant and suddenly the neurotic woman who was unable to cope with anything vanished into thin air. I had a complicated pregnancy and a difficult baby and I coped perfectly. My boyfriend even walked out on me and I still carried on coping. Such a thing had previously been unimaginable. I was a woman who spent two weeks of each month in total shock, as if I was recovering from a major trauma.

The third week I would be suicidal – I attempted to kill

myself on several occasions. I took overdoses, cut myself, and even poured boiling water over my body. Once, I remember thinking, 'Funny, that . . . I always seem to have my period when I'm in hospital!' I didn't realize that I was only in hospital *because* I was having my period!

Only the fourth week of my cycle was good enough that I felt I could take on the world.

Then, during the 18 months of pregnancy and early motherhood when I wasn't menstruating, I realized there had to be a connection between not having periods and being able to cope with whatever life threw at me.

My loony behaviour started when my periods started . . . and stopped when they stopped. I was over the moon when I realized I'd found the answer. The problem was, how to convince a doctor that my problems were all due to PMS?

Many doctors claim that teenagers are too young to suffer from PMS. But, as Fiona's story testifies, it can actually start with the first period. This is, after all, a time of great hormonal change. Fortunately, Fiona's example is unusual and many women do not get PMS until much later in their life. And those who do get it as teenagers usually develop the first symptoms two to three years after the onset of menstruation.

Jane's story shows how problems can start during use of the Pill.

I'd been on the Pill since the age of 18 and had used the same one – Ovulin 50 – right up to the age of 26. I was perfectly content with it. It felt safe and caused no side-effects. But, during one of my routine visits to my doctor, I was told I was now too old for Ovulin 50 and should change to a new Pill. It was around the time that there was a lot of fuss about giving high-oestrogen pills to women over 25 and, although I was surprised that I was going to have to change, I didn't question my doctor's decision. In fact, I felt pleased that he was taking such good care of me.

He suggested I tried Conova 30, which had a lower oestrogen level, and that sounded fine to me.

I should point out that, up until this time, I had never experienced anything that I could associate with PMS. Neither on the Pill nor before I had started taking it in my teens.

But, within a few weeks of starting on Conova 30, I became aware of a very slight difference in myself. I couldn't put my finger on it, but I knew I just wasn't normal.

The doctor accepted that maybe the Conova 30 wasn't agreeing with me, but he couldn't put me back on Ovulin 50, and suggested I tried one of the new Minipills instead.

I still didn't go back to my normal old self, but I persevered with the Minipill.

I was working in the film industry at the time, and I remember one lunchtime sitting in the bar and suddenly feeling that I was going to pass out. Looking back, I think it was a low blood sugar attack and probably the first really dramatic symptom of PMS I'd ever had.

My secretary later said that I often used to complain about funny moments and she noticed it was always in the week before my period.

Then, after an unplanned pregnancy and abortion in 1988, I came off the Pill and had a coil fitted. My PMS didn't get any worse, but it didn't improve either. I continued having near-fainting attacks, followed by fits of aggression and panic.

It was only when I finally had the coil removed, 18 months ago, that my PMS disappeared for good. I remember looking in my diary, six months after it was taken out, and thinking, 'That's amazing! I've got rid of my PMS!' I could only think that, somehow, the removal of my coil had jolted my system back to normal!

Dr Katharina Dalton points out that women who suffer from PMS are liable to experience side-effects when they are on the Pill, and that the IUD (coil) can cause increased oestrogen production, resulting, in some women, in a hormone imbalance.

Even in women who have never previously suffered from PMS, coming off the Pill can bring about symptoms for the first time. The Pill contains a manmade steroid called progestogen, which acts as a contraceptive and also lowers the level of progesterone in the blood. This means the Pill produces a progesterone deficiency in those women whose normal progesterone production is not flexible enough to counteract the action of the progestogen.

Jackie's story shows how stress can cause PMS.

I had never been aware of suffering from PMS until I was approaching my fortieth birthday and my two children were entering their teens.

Then, slowly, over a period of two years I noticed certain changes. The worst was an increasing awareness that I had bad breath, but I also suffered irritability and headaches.

I'd had my teeth checked by my dentist and I knew that there was nothing wrong in that department which was causing my halitosis. It was only when my headaches and irritability became so severe that I sought outside help, that I realized my bad breath was another symptom of PMS and was caused by pasties that I was craving.

I am convinced my PMS came on when it did because of stress in my life.

My son had had open heart surgery when he was a toddler, and the doctors had warned me that he may need another operation when he reached his teens. Throughout his childhood I'd been able to put all thoughts about this to the back of my mind, but, once he reached 13, I couldn't help worrying myself sick about him.

Stress predisposes us to PMS. Even when we are not totally aware that we are under stress, underlying anxieties can trigger the onset of symptoms.

Kate's story shows how having a child can bring about changes that cause PMS.

I used to be one of those irritating women who claim they never have PMS and never even know when their period is due. I was on an even keel for the whole month, and felt exasperated by friends who blamed emotional outbursts on their hormones.

Then I had my daughter, and everything changed. I became very snappy and tearful – and put the blame on the stress of being a working mother. As my little girl grew into a toddler, I'd ache with guilt after shouting at her over something trivial. But I felt so engulfed with rage that I thought I was going to roar like a lion or shake her to her senses. After an outburst, I'd tremble with shock, my face set rigid with tension. And I'd become depressed and weepy and tell myself I had to be the worst mother in the world.

That would lead me to thinking what a pitiful and useless person I was, not just as a mother but as a wife, a friend and a worker. And I'd feel so low, that I imagined everyone else was saying the same thing about me, that I was a complete waste of space . . . The following week, however, I would be buoyant, gregarious, my daughter's best friend and she would reward me with big kisses and cards telling me how much she loved me.

It took me years, though, to realize that a change had come about when I'd had her and, much as I hated to admit it, I now suffered from PMS. I wasn't a bad mother at all – those outbursts were few and far between, though, magnified, they made me feel like a monster. And I wasn't a pitiful person or a waste of space. I was just a normal woman with normal monthly symptoms and I would just have to accept that and do something about it if I could.

You might develop PMS for the first time after your first, second of even third baby. If this happens, one explanation as to why is that you are more vulnerable than others to hormonal changes and so your hormonal system never clicks back in place after a birth.

Dr Dalton also points out that during pregnancy, higher levels of progesterone than normal are continually present in the blood for nine months and not just two weeks at a time as in non-pregnant women. During the early weeks of pregnancy, this extra progesterone is produced by the ovary and as the placenta (afterbirth) develops in the womb it becomes a progesterone factory, producing greater and greater amounts of the hormone. During labour, after the baby is born, the placenta or progesterone factory comes away and some women have difficulty in adjusting again to producing sufficient progesterone. It is these who develop PMS.

Theresa's story shows how PMS can occur as you grow older.

I don't remember ever having problems of any kind with my periods before the age of 30. But, since then, my symptoms have become more intense by the year.

I put this down to two factors: firstly that, as we grow older, our hormones become more turbulent; secondly, that, since 30, I have had more stress in my life.

Between the ages of 35 and 40 I had problems at work, a troubled marriage, and a Rackman-like landlord. And I definitely noticed that the level of stress in my life at any one time had a direct bearing on the intensity of my PMS.

If I was on holiday, I could go through a month at a time with no symptoms. I even spent one whole year in Australia with my family and never knew when my period was due.

Now, at 40, I can feel my PMS stretching beyond the usual one bad week. I feel tetchy, bloated and very sensitive to what people say for two to three weeks every month. And I have also noticed that my figure takes longer to go back to its normal size after my period. Once, I could count on being slim within a couple of days of the onset of bleeding. Now, I seem to be bulky for most of the month – either because my period is approaching or because I am recovering from it.

PMS can become a worsening problem as you approach menopause which, typically, takes place between the ages of 45 and 50. PMS starting late in life, before the age of 45, frequently continues until menopause if it is left untreated.

Susan's story shows how PMS can start as a result of dietary factors.

> I'd always been a skinny child and found it difficult to accept the new curves I developed in my teens. I wanted to remain rake-like and, at the age of 18, I started dieting.
>
> I'd skip breakfast, then go as long as I could during the day without eating anything. Then, at teatime, I'd fill up on cakes and crisps. I ended up fatter than ever, but also grumpy, tearful and unable to cope well with life during my premenstrual phase.

Slimming diets are often begun in the premenstrual phase when we feel particularly dissatisfied with our body shape and when depression and heightened sensitivity to criticism make us feel we should be making a bigger effort to look good. But drastic diets in the premenstrual phase are likely to be followed by binges. The teenage years can be a time when bad eating habits set in for life, and serve to aggravate the cause and symptoms of PMS. A healthy, balanced diet may help relieve your PMS, but may take many months before it begins to work.

If you are considering dieting, see Chapter 6 for tips on losing weight while eating sensibly to counteract symptoms. Also, try to resist starting your diet before your period as this is a time when many of us are tempted to overeat anyway. If you start a new diet at the beginning of a cycle, you will, hopefully, have had time to get used to some of your new eating habits when your premenstrual phase starts. And you will feel better about the way you look when you start the diet.

4

Getting a diagnosis

Pamela was in her late thirties when she went to the doctor about her PMS.

> I was getting severe migraines every month. The pain was so bad that it would shoot down the left-hand side of my body, penetrating my arm, back and leg. But when I told my doctor I thought it was to do with PMT (as we knew it in those days) he said, 'Well, in that case, you can rest assured that it's not life-threatening.' He told me to take a painkiller and try to forget about it. He wasn't interested in treating it any further.

That was 20 years ago. Most of us would expect a more sympathetic response these days, but don't bank on it!

Although some GPs have a special interest in PMS, most do not. Their job is to treat the 'presenting' illness. If you consult your doctor about a rash, he or she will look at treating your spots. If backache is troubling you, he or she will prescribe something to alleviate the pain. If it is persistent, he or she may refer you to a physiotherapist. He or she will often not make the connection with PMS, unless you give good reasons. It is therefore vital that you give your doctor as much information as you possibly can to get the most accurate diagnosis and treatment.

Fiona told us in the last chapter how, after having her baby, she realized that her normally bizarre and incapable behaviour must have been due to PMS. Until then, doctors had been treating her for depression.

> When my periods returned – along with the accompanying PMS – after the birth of my little boy, I felt I had to prove to my GP that the problem was premenstrual.
>
> I had been keeping a diary and looking back through it for

clues about the pattern of my behaviour made horrific reading. Just looking at it, not even reading, I could see the change in myself. My writing is normally very neat, but prior to my period, it was large, loopy, erratic and angry-looking.

I had recently moved areas, so I felt I was going to my new doctor with a clean slate. She was the first GP who had ever even considered that the problem could be PMS. She said there was only one way to find out for sure, and that was to stop my periods artificially. She prescribed a steroid spray called buseralin, which suppressed my periods and stopped my PMS.

If I could have stayed on the buseralin for ever, my problems would have been over because it certainly did the trick for my PMS. But buseralin can only be used short term, so the symptoms would have to be treated by other means.

Finding a treatment that suited me actually proved a great problem. But I was happy that at least I had found a doctor who was on my side and willing to help me find what I needed. It was a good starting point.

Keep a diary

If you suspect your problems are associated with PMS, and are serious about getting the treatment you need, you may, like Fiona, have to prove your case to your GP. One way of doing this is to invest in a spacious diary and, over the course of three months, keep a daily note of:

- your emotions, that is, irritable, weepy, depressed or whatever (even if you do not feel that your emotions are noteworthy, do record any upsets or arguments you have had and the subject of them – 'cashier rude to me in Sainsbury's' or 'furious with children for being late getting up for school' – as they may later translate as a big fuss over nothing but the fact that they occurred is important)
- any physical symptoms, such as headache, nausea, bloating, sore breasts, fatigue, spottiness, mouth ulcers

- what you ate, for example, 'breakfast: coffee, toast, butter, jam; lunch: cheese and tomato sandwich; supper: spaghetti bolognese and salad'
- what you drank – try to keep a record of fluids consumed, say, a.m.: three cups of coffee; lunch: Coke; p.m.: three cups of tea; evening· two glasses of red wine
- any exercise you took, say, 'walked the dog, cycled to the shops, swimming class in evening' (and if you didn't leave the house, say so – be honest with your diary because it's for your own good)
- any current stress or worries in your life, for example, 'worried about money today'; 'a lot of work on, late leaving the office'.

Keep a separate chart

At the end of each week, on a separate monthly chart, make a note of the main physical and emotional symptoms you have suffered, and also when your period started and finished.

Charting symptoms is an important key to diagnosis as it provides an at-a-glance picture of *when* the symptoms occur during the menstrual cycle, which symptoms are linked to the *cycle* and which are present at *other* times, too. Invariably women who keep a chart realize that some of the symptoms they thought were premenstrual actually occurred through the whole month, while symptoms they did not associate with PMS are, in fact, surprisingly relevant.

Don't look on your diary keeping and charting as a chore. Together, they will help you identify precisely when and how you are experiencing PMS. The notes about diet and exercise may also give you clues for how best to alleviate some of the problems.

At the end of three months, a pattern to your symptoms will have emerged and, by transferring your notes from your diary to your chart, you will be able to pick out this pattern very clearly.

Take your chart, and even your diary, with you when you go to see your doctor for a diagnosis.

Is your doctor willing to help?

Medical practitioners may be less informed about PMS than the patient who has read articles and books on the subject. This doesn't matter too much, as long as the doctor you see is prepared to listen to what you have to say and to consider your problem seriously.

Nicky was at rock-bottom with PMS and had left home to live with her mother. She says:

> My mother's GP was marvellous! He admitted he didn't know much about PMS, but that obviously I did and he could certainly see the logic of what I was saying. He helped me get the treatment I needed, after years of failure with other doctors, and he even invited me back to the surgery, a year ago, to give a talk on PMS and its treatment.

Arrange an appointment with your GP during the 'good' week or fortnight of your cycle. Do not see the doctor when you are premenstrual, because, although you are *experiencing* the symptoms at that time, you also risk becoming irrational, argumentative, oversensitive or snappy if the doctor seems unsympathetic.

Take your diary and charts with you, and explain, as clearly as possible, why you think your symptoms may be linked to PMS.

In medical training, 'women's troubles' are often the butt of teaching jokes. Doctors get used to ignoring them, laughing at them and discounting them. By making an appointment during your rational time of the month and showing your doctor that you have already taken steps (with your diary and charts) to identify your problem for yourself, you will prove that you are serious about it. It is not something that is bothering you today and will be forgotten tomorrow.

Don't be embarrassed about consulting your doctor about PMS. A lot of women feel this is something they should learn to put up with and that they are wasting their doctor's time by booking an appointment.

Julie, a 35-year-old mother, says she'd noticed her PMS get considerably worse after the birth of her daughter.

I became very quick to fly off the handle. Molehills became mountains and I was tense, irritable, very depressed and craved sugary, sweet foods. But I never got round to booking myself an appointment with my GP. Instead I asked about it while I was in the surgery about something to do with my little girl. It was teatime. He was running late. I had already asked about three small things and it was just sort of chipped in at the last minute. No sooner had I spat out the word 'premenstrual' than he was writing me a prescription for vitamin B$_6$, and that was that! I really didn't feel he was the slightest bit interested in treating *my* PMS as opposed to PMS in general.

By cheating yourself of a full consultation, you will come away, as Julie did, feeling that you haven't been taken seriously. Treat yourself to the time you would demand if you thought one of your children was ill. (If necessary, tell yourself the whole family will benefit if you're treated!)

Ask your practitioner questions that will tell you a bit about his or her attitude to your problem, such as the following.

- What causes PMS? The way in which your doctor answers this will show you how interested he or she is.
- What are the possible treatments for it? Look for variety in the suggestions offered.
- Which therapies has the doctor used and why?
- What is your doctor's favourite form of treatment?
- What are the risks of each treatment?
- What are the costs of each treatment? (In some cases, an expensive treatment may not be prescribed if the doctor thinks it will break his or her budget.)

Equally, there are questions your doctor should ask you. Your GP will be showing a genuine and serious interest in your complaint if he or she asks for:

- a list of symptoms and when they appear
- details of your menstrual pattern
- your gynaecological, obstetric and contraceptive history.

Your doctor will also want to ask the following questions.

- Did the symptoms appear for the first time after a change of contraceptive method?
- Did they start after childbirth?
- Did you have postnatal depression?
- How long have your symptoms been troubling you?
- Have you tried any self-help therapies? / are you willing to try these?
- Have there been any major changes in your life recently?
- What is your general lifestyle like? How much stress do you have? What is your diet like and how much exercise do you take?
- Have you any other physical symptoms that you do not associate with PMS?

If you are *not* asked these questions, volunteer the information anyway. Your diary and charts will have given you most of the answers you need and you should feel well clued up on the precise nature of your own PMS when you see your doctor.

The doctor may also want to give you an internal examination, to rule out any other causes of your symptoms, such as endometriosis.

Your own attitudes will partly influence the way your doctor treats you. This is a problem if you are worried your doctor won't believe you. For a lot of women, coming to terms with PMS involves at least one consultation with an unhelpful doctor. If this happens to you, put it down to experience, but *don't* give up. And don't put up with any treatment that you feel is less than adequate. Shop around long enough and you will find a doctor (or alternative practitioner) you know you can work with.

5

What your doctor can do for you

Having identified the pattern and symptoms of your PMS, you may, by this stage, have already reached the conclusion that a self-help approach will be better for you than medical intervention.

Even if this is the case, I would recommend at least one trip to your GP – with your diaries and charts – so that PMS can be confirmed and any more serious condition can be ruled out.

Unless your symptoms are extremely severe, your doctor may also suggest self-help treatments as a first resort. These include vitamins, minerals and evening primrose oil (all of which may be offered on prescription) and a change to your eating habits and exercise routine.

As a general rule, though, remember that there is no single magic treatment that works for everyone. Indeed, the process of finding the right treatment for you may be a long one. You may start off with vitamin supplements and end up with progesterone suppositories. Better this way round than starting with medication that is unnecessary, however.

PMS can be stubborn, too. One treatment may appear to be working for a while, then, lo and behold, the Jekyll and Hyde symptoms return. Also, *total* relief from symptoms may be hard to achieve, but then major relief from them is a godsend!

If you have found a doctor who is willing to listen to what you are telling him or her, and is keen to help, be patient. Cracking the jigsaw puzzle is as much a problem for the doctor as it is for you.

Forgetting for the moment the self-help remedies the doctor may suggest, and which we will be returning to in the next chapter, let's look at the medical options a GP can offer.

These include hormonal treatments, antiprostaglandins, diuretics, antidepressants and tranquillizers. However, because PMS is still so badly understood by a great number of doctors,

52

the medical treatments suggested may not always be those that an expert in PMS would recommend.

Hormonal treatments

The Pill

What is it?

There are many contraceptive pills available on prescription. Most combine progestogen and oestrogen. The Pill serves to increase natural hormonal levels in the body, interfering with the production of FSH and LH in the pituitary gland and preventing ovulation from taking place, thereby preventing pregnancy.

Why is it prescribed for PMS?

The Pill is often prescribed because it levels out the naturally occurring peaks and troughs of our monthly hormonal changes and protects us from swings towards too much or too little oestrogen or progesterone. However:

- a small number of women continue to suffer symptoms of PMS while on the Pill, which suggests that the Pill does not completely suppress hormonal changes
- the Pill has its own unpleasant side-effects for some women – and one of these is depression, so you could find yourself jumping out of the frying pan and into the fire
- women who have never suffered from PMS while on the Pill have, however, discovered the syndrome for the first time coming off it (according to research by Katharina Dalton, this is because the Pill contains the manmade steroid called progestogen, which mimics progesterone, but actually has the effect of lowering natural progesterone levels, which means that the Pill produces a progesterone deficiency in some women).

Danazol

What is it?

Danazol is a drug often used to treat endometriosis (where some of the tissue lining the uterus – endometrium – grows in other parts of the body, usually the pelvic area) and menorrhagia (abnormally heavy periods). By suppressing the release of LH and FSH it reduces the production and release of oestrogen from the ovaries. The change in hormone levels usually prevents ovulation and results in irregularity or complete absence of menstruation.

Why is it prescribed for PMS?

The effects of danazol on the ovaries is to suppress the hormonal highs and lows we would otherwise experience, along with their PMS side-effects. However:

- adverse effects may include nausea, dizziness, rashes, back pain, weight gain and flushes, which many women claim are worse than the original symptoms of PMS.

Note that pregnancy should be avoided if you are taking danazol because it can cause masculine characteristics in a female foetus.

Bromocriptine

What is it?

Bromocriptine is a drug that dampens down production of the hormone prolactin by the anterior pituitary gland. It is used to treat abnormal milk production by the breast and some types of male and female infertility. New mothers who do not wish to breastfeed may also be given bromocriptine. It is also used in the treatment of Parkinson's disease, as it is very similar to dopamine, the chemical lacking in the brains of people with Parkinson's.

Why is it prescribed for PMS?

Women whose main symptom of PMS is severe premenstrual breast discomfort may be helped by taking bromocriptine.

However, adverse effects include vomiting and nausea, and very high doses can cause drowsiness and confusion.

Progestogen pills

What are they?

Progestogens are an artificial form of progesterone. They are a component of the Pill and are also used in hormone replacement therapy in combination with an oestrogen drug to protect against the risk of cancer of the uterus, which may occur if oestrogens alone are taken over a long period of time.

Why are they prescribed for PMS?

Doctors prescribe progestogens thinking they do the same thing as natural progesterone, and they are easier to administer as they can be taken orally (natural progesterone cannot). They have some progesterone-like actions, but they can actually make PMS worse – hence the lack of enthusiasm among doctors for natural progesterone, which they confuse with progestogen.

The adverse effects include weight gain, oedema (water retention), loss of appetite, headache, dizziness, rashes, irregular periods, breast tenderness, and, rarely, ovarian cysts.

Natural progesterone

What is it?

Progesterone is the female sex hormone that ensures the smooth running of the female reproductive system. It is produced by the ovaries during the second half of the menstrual cycle and by the placenta during pregnancy.

The progesterone given as a treatment for PMS is derived from an extract of the root of the yam vegetable.

Why is it prescribed for PMS?

Natural progesterone boosts flagging progesterone levels, which are often the cause of PMS. The treatment was pioneered by Dr Katharina Dalton and it has so far helped thousands of women for whom other treatments have failed.

Progesterone cannot be absorbed orally and must, therefore, be administered by means of vaginal or rectal suppositories, or, for very severe cases, via deep intramuscular injections.

When progesterone works well, it provides immediate relief – within an hour. However, it sometimes only gives slight relief, in which case larger doses may be required (some doctors give women the choice of a normal 'three a day dose' or 'four a day' for bad days).

There are a few important points to remember that will enhance your likelihood of success with progesterone:

- time rectal suppositories so their absorption is not prevented by a stool in the rectum
- progesterone therapy can sometimes take months to work because of the need to adjust the timing and dose to suit the symptoms which may vary from cycle to cycle
- if you have a very short, symptom-free time each month, you may find yourself taking progesterone all month (the major difficulty with this is that constant progesterone use can cause spotting and bleeding throughout your cycle)
- feeling sleepy, confused or lethargic can be a sign that you are taking too much progesterone
- the range in doses of progesterone prescribed for PMS is enormous – anything from 200 to 4000 mg daily.

Common questions about progesterone therapy

Q How long will I have to continue with therapy?

A Some women use progesterone for many years. Others experience such relief after one or two years that they are able to come off treatment altogether. Unfortunately, there is no way of telling in advance who will need long-term and who will benefit from short-term treatment.

Q Are there any side-effects?

A Unpleasant side-effects are very unusual, but slight spotting or bleeding through the month may occur if you are using progesterone for most of your cycle. Suppositories may also cause some breast tenderness, early or late periods, increased menstrual cramps, decreased libido, faintness, headaches and vaginal yeast infections (thrush). These sound pretty horrendous, but are unlikely to be as severe as when they are symptoms of PMS. Injections can bring on the reactions in some women, as well as the possibility of abscesses at the site of the injection. Injections are painful, but if you are unable to absorb progesterone via suppositories they may be worth a try.

Q Is it safe to use progesterone therapy prior to trying to become pregnant?

A No. Do not use progesterone during the cycles in which you plan to conceive. Although it is unlikely to harm your baby, no controlled studies have looked at the effects of progesterone on the unborn child, and it is really a case of better safe than sorry. If you discover you are pregnant, stop taking progesterone immediately. However, if you are planning a pregnancy in the next few months, there is no need to give up treatment until the cycle in which you plan to conceive. Progesterone is almost entirely excreted by the body within a day or two of taking it, so progesterone from past cycles will not hang around.

Oestradiol implants

What are they?

These are one of the newest and most controversial of the hormone treatments available for PMS. Their use has been pioneered by John Studd, who runs a PMS clinic at the Dulwich Hospital in London.

Oestradiol is a synthetic form of the hormone oestrogen and is also used to treat symptoms and complications of the menopause.

Some women complain of severe side-effects with oestradiol, which include breast pain, nausea, weight gain and headaches.

Antiprostaglandins

What are they?

Prostaglandins are substances manufactured by our bodies. They are responsible for making us feel pain and inflammation and can cause excessive contractions of the uterus, stomach, intestines and so on. Antiprostaglandins counter the effects of pro-staglandins.

Why are they prescribed for PMS?

Antiprostaglandin drugs, which include aspirin and Nurofen, may be prescribed to relieve physical symptoms of PMS, such as cramps, headaches, bloating, nausea and breast pain.

Antidepressants

What are they?

Antidepressant drugs are used in the treatment of depression and work either by triggering the release of chemicals in the brain to stimulate nerve activity or by prolonging the life of these chemicals after their release.

The main types of antidepressants are:

- tricyclics, which have a sedative effect; side-effects include constipation, digestive problems, heart palpitations and difficulty reaching orgasm, to name but a few
- mao inhibitors, which are stronger than tricyclics; side-effects include agitation, confusion and hallucinations and they react badly with certain foods, such as cheese, chicken livers, yeast and citrus fruits
- lithium salts, which are fairly controversial, coming in and out of favour with doctors, and usually prescribed for manic depressive illness.

Note that antidepressants tend to interact with other drugs so you should always check with your doctor before combining antidepressants with any other medication.

Why are they prescribed for PMS?

Antidepressants are frequently prescribed, but, unless depression is the *only* severe symptom of PMS you suffer from they are unlikely to be of very much benefit.

Diuretics

What are they?

This is a group of drugs used to gather excess water from around the body and remove it in the form of urine. They work by interfering with the normal filtration process of the kidneys and either reduce the amount of water taken back into the bloodstream (and hence around the body) or increase the blood flow through the kidneys and thus the amount of water they filter and expel in the urine.

Why are they prescribed for PMS?

Diuretics are widely used for PMS, despite the fact that they have little effect on relieving the symptoms! Although they remove fluid from the body, they can also increase lethargy and just generally feeling awful.

Other side-effects include weakness, confusion and palpitations. Some diuretic drugs can increase the risk of gout or cause or aggravate diabetes mellitus.

Tranquillizers

What are they?

Tranquillizers are drugs that have a sedative effect. There are two main types: antipsychotic drugs and antianxiety drugs.

Antipsychotic drugs are normally used to treat schizophrenia and manic depressive illness and they work by blocking the action of dopamine, a chemical that stimulates nerve activity in the brain.

Antianxiety drugs are used to provide temporary relief from anxiety when it limits a patient's ability to cope with everyday life. They promote mental and physical relaxation by reducing nerve activity in the brain.

Why are they prescribed for PMS?

Tranquillizers tend to be prescribed when the doctor prescribing them is either unaware that the patient is suffering from PMS or he or she cannot think what else to do.

The problem is that although tranquillizers help to relieve intense irritability and violent outbursts, they also damp down a number of functions in the brain, including the centres where emotions are experienced, and this results in depression – one of the commonest problems PMS sufferers are trying to escape from!

Tranquillizers are also highly addictive and should be kept for short-term emergency use only – and preferably not at all for PMS. If your GP suggests tranquillizers, ask for something else!

Other treatments

Remember PMS is still a relatively new area of medicine. It is also a confusing one – for doctors as well as patients. Symptoms of PMS can look like symptoms of other complaints, too. Success with different treatments varies from one woman to another, and it can be difficult for a GP to know exactly what to do.

Be prepared, as mentioned earlier, to put an unhelpful doctor down to experience. Persevere and you will, eventually, find the help you need.

This said, the following are to be avoided if at all possible:

- hysterectomy – this has often been prescribed, but found to make PMS worse as general depression can follow a hysterectomy and, unless the ovaries are also removed, the cycle of PMS also continues

- Provera and Depo-Provera are long-acting progestogens sometimes given by injection to stop ovulation and periods for a few months, but they can cause depression and it can take months to get the drug out of your system. So, if your doctor says you are getting progesterone tablets, beware – progesterone, as we have already noted, does *not* come in tablet form; Provera and Depo-Provera *do*
- electroconvulsive therapy (ECT), or shock treatment, is a radical and very controversial treatment sometimes used for PMS, but it has very serious long-term consequences, including effects on the memory and thinking ability, and it has not been shown to be of any use in treating PMS.

Personal experiences

Members of The Aberdeen Premenstrual Support Group were asked, 'Have you contacted anyone about your PMS? If so, what did he/she say?' Here are a few of their replies.

My doctor told me that if I felt Evening Primrose Oil was helping, I could use that. But he didn't offer me any other information or advice.

My GP gave me a chart to monitor my symptoms for a few months.

My doctor prescribed tablets, but I didn't want to take them! So the pill bottle remained unopened on my dressing table.

My doctor was no help at all.

When I spoke to my GP, he remained completely silent. Didn't have a thing to say to me!

I went to my doctor (twice). He just listened to me and it was a relief just to be able to tell someone how I felt.

My lady doctor said it was hard to tell if it was PMS.

My doctor told me to write down everything I felt during the week leading up to my period.

My doctor prescribed diuretics three years ago. They helped with the bloating, but I didn't stay on them long term.

My doctor was extremely helpful and supplied various treatments and loads of advice.

As these responses show, every doctor and every woman's experience with her doctor will be different. Some GPs are sceptical about PMS, but others are not. Don't give up!

Here is Joyce's story.

I had suffered for years from PMS and knew all the signs, but I only finally went to my doctor about it two years ago.

I didn't want to mess around, and I wanted to show him I knew what I was talking about. So, for three months before seeing him, I kept a chart of my cycle, marking my period with an X, and noting any symptoms as they occurred.

The first symptom was always an irresistible craving for chocolate and caramel sweets 10 days before my period. That would last for two or three days. Then I would become bad-tempered and violent, clumsy and forgetful.

I'd drop things for no apparent reason – one minute a glass would be in my hands, the next it would be in smithereens on the floor. I'd say something to somebody, then repeat myself word for word two minutes later. I was hopeless! My breasts were also extremely sore and heavy and I couldn't bear to be touched because even brushing against someone was agony.

I told my GP how I felt, showed him the charts and explained that I'd already tried evening primrose oil and a high carbohydrate diet, but neither had been very successful.

As I particularly wanted to lose weight, I found it hard to eat several small meals a day without piling on the pounds. And I thought there must be something else my GP could suggest.

He listened really well and was extremely sympathetic. I felt I could have poured my heart out to him all afternoon and he wouldn't have tried to turn me away.

Finally he said, 'You're describing your problem very well. It is PMS and there are three things we can try as a first resort.'

These were evening primrose oil – but, as I've said, I'd already tried that and abandoned it – tranquillizers – but I wasn't interested in those, they only mask your feelings instead of helping you to deal with them – and, lastly, vitamin B_6.

Well, somewhere at the back of my mind I remembered having tried vitamin B_6, but had given it up because of the cost. I didn't realize you could also get it on prescription from your GP. So I agreed to give it another go.

Had I gone back three months later complaining that the vitamins had done no good, I'm sure my doctor would have helped me find something else. But we didn't get that far, because, for me, vitamin B_6 turned out to be the perfect solution.

I am now on a regular repeat prescription. I start on the tablets on day 14 of my cycle and, within a day, my breasts are comfortable and my moods are manageable. My dose is 50 mg twice a day until day two or three of my new cycle.

I'm so grateful to my doctor for taking me seriously and giving me the help I needed. I don't know what I would have done without him!

Here is Jackie's story.

Ever since I started my periods, at the age of 15, I've had to go to bed with flu-like exhaustion for two days every month before my period. But it wasn't until I went through a major trauma (my uncle and aunt both died and my father became ill with skin cancer), two years ago, that my symptoms became so bad I realized it must be PMS.

I'm not normally a moaning minnie, and I'd only been to my GP once in the last three years (for what he called post-viral flu, which I now realize must also have been PMS), but when I told him I was convinced I was suffering from PMS, he instantly dismissed the idea.

The first thing he asked was, 'How old are you?' When I told him I was 45, he said, 'Well, that's it then: you're menopausal!' That threw me completely, but I didn't like to argue.

He said, 'Any hot flushes?'

'No!', I said.

'What about scanty periods?', he asked.

'No,' I said, 'They're normal too!'

He hummed and hawed – I had none of the symptoms of menopause, but he honestly didn't know what else to do with me. He didn't know enough about PMS to realize that the diagnosis I had arrived at was actually the right one.

He put me straight onto Prempak-C Hormone Replacement Therapy, which is used for menopausal women and which provides doses of oestrogen and progestogen (a synthetic form of progesterone) in cycles. I was fine on the oestrogen. But the minute I started on the progestogens, my whole system went wild – I had every menopausal and PMS symptom in the book!

I've since discovered I have a progesterone deficiency and the artificial progestogen was making this worse by blocking my progesterone receptors and preventing the little progesterone I was producing from getting through.

Everything went off-course after that. Unfortunately, my doctor did all the wrong things. He'd started me on HRT (which I didn't need) in the middle of my cycle (it should start at the beginning, if at all). I then suffered a heavy mid-month bleed and he sent me off for a D and C (dilation and curettage, a procedure in which the lining of the womb is scraped away, but which is known – trust my luck – to aggravate PMS!). And, when I was still no better, he sent me back to the consultant gynaecologist who put me on, horror of horrors, double doses of HRT oestrogen patches, which further exacerbated the imbalance between my progesterone and oestrogen levels!

Mine is a horror story, I know, but a lot of women have had similar experiences and I want to prevent others from going through the same thing.

In the end I couldn't walk, I couldn't sleep, I was scared to go out because I thought I'd have panic attacks, but I felt trapped if I stayed in. My life was hell. And my beautiful home was like a prison.

I've always been very well off and have led a happy, comfortable life, but I felt then that no amount of wealth could compensate for ill-health.

Normally I'm the type of woman who's running around doing keep-fit, holding dinner parties and working hard with the family business, but I was so ill that I couldn't even bring myself to sort through a basket of laundry without bursting into tears and putting myself to bed.

My GP called in a psychologist who said I was depressed. He put me on tranquillizers and antidepressants (all alongside the HRT I was still battling away with). But, impossible though it seemed at this stage, they made me even worse!

I've since discovered that the tricyclic antidepressants he prescribed had the effect of reducing prolactin levels, which in turn lower progesterone levels – everything was against me!

Suspecting that the drugs were making me worse, I phoned a good friend who's a biochemist. She listened to me listing the ingredients of the drug cocktail I was taking and tutted. 'You should never be taking that lot together!', she said. 'Now promise me you're going to be very brave and chuck all those antidepressants and tranquillizers down the loo.'

I promised and did it straight away. But the depression continued and my psychologist eventually told me he thought I was having a nervous breakdown.

'No way!', I said, 'I'm sure it's not that!' I phoned my husband to come home early and he actually arrived with his brother.

I remember my brother-in-law, who's a farmer, took one look at me and said, 'Are you on something? I've seen sheep act the way you're acting!'

'Oh, thanks a bunch!', I said.

'No, I mean it,' he said, 'sheep who're on hormones . . . are you taking something?'

At the back of my mind I'd known it for a long time, but hearing it from my brother-in-law convinced me that the HRT was responsible for my illness.

I am not a religious person, but that night, I swear, God stepped in and saved me. My sister-in-law said I needed help immediately and she picked up the phone there and then and called the local Well Woman Clinic in Canterbury.

The next day I had an appointment with a brilliant lady doctor.

I remember saying to her as I arrived, 'My psychologist thinks I'm having a nervous breakdown!'

'No,' she said, 'you're not having a breakdown! But you've got a terrific hormone imbalance.' She asked me about my cravings. They were all for acidic foods, like pickled onions – and I'd craved exactly the same things when I was pregnant. She said, 'It looks like your hormones are all over the place!'

She took me off all the treatments I was on – HRT, tranquillizers, the lot.

'This is going to be difficult,' she said, 'but for three months you're going to give your system a rest – let it get rid of all the old medication – and you're going to chart your diet, emotions and symptoms.'

Three months later, she wrote to my GP asking him to put me on Cyclogest – progesterone suppositories.

These cost £1 a shot, and not every GP wants to prescribe them.

When I saw my GP, he asked why I'd gone to the Well Woman Clinic. I didn't want to be too snappy with him, but I couldn't stop myself from saying: 'You've got me in this mess, they're going to get me out of it!'

He huffed and puffed and said, 'Well, I've never known anyone have any success with progesterone.' I said, 'Well, let's just try it and see, shall we?'

I was determined to make an impression when I went back for my second prescription, three months later. I did my hair, dressed smartly. Made sure my make-up was immaculate. I felt great, and I wanted it to show.

He was noticeably impressed! He couldn't stop looking at me as he wrote out the prescription. And when we began to talk about it, I realized he'd done his homework and had found out a bit about PMS – not before time!

I'd been so angry with him earlier on for letting me down. But now, looking at him, I felt sorry for him. How many women, I wondered, had walked into his practice expecting help for their PMS and been fobbed off with the wrong treatment. He honestly hadn't known what to do until I came along with my letter asking for progesterone.

What is frightening, though, is that a lot of women don't get the treatment they need and they don't realize that you can make an appointment with a Well Woman Clinic without a doctor's referral. Let my experience be of encouragement to others.

6

What you can do for yourself –
self-help for PMS

Louise is 29 years old and single. Her periods started early, when she was 11 years old, and she remembers the first signs of PMS creeping up on her when she was 15 or 16.

To be honest, the earlier years are quite vague. I'd always have some pain – cramp or wind, which was distinct from period pain – the day before my period started.

But, as I got older, I developed more severe symptoms and began to notice a pattern to them.

It would start with a high – I'd be extremely bouncy and energetic. Then, the next day, boom! My irritability and crippling cramps would set in. I was very emotional, tearful and completely irrational. I thought I was the only woman in the world who suffered the way I did.

People used to make jokes about PMS – 'Oh, don't take any notice of Louise, it's just her time of the month!' That kind of thing. I used to think, 'Is that supposed to be funny?' I don't find it funny. Why do we joke about PMS instead of treating it?

My behaviour was very bad premenstrually and I soon found I could get away with being rude, late and so on by using my PMS as an excuse.

After a while, I got so used to using PMS as an excuse that I couldn't distinguish between the premenstrual behaviour and bad behaviour in general. I started to think I must be mad – and eventually realized that I had to identify PMS one way or the other.

My doctor put me on the Pill, but I didn't take to it very well. It made me feel sick, and I disliked the flow of blood it produced as a mock period. It was more like gunge than true blood flow.

I also didn't like the idea of it. It made me uneasy to think of something interfering with my body the way the Pill did.

So I came off it, and tried another drug. The doctor had recommended Ponstan, which is an antiprostaglandin muscle relaxant, often used for period pains.

Again, I had a problem coming to terms with the idea of taking a drug – and, quite honestly, it didn't seem to be any more effective than a common or garden Anadin.

I wanted something which was natural and non-invasive, so I arranged to see a yogic counsellor. Her name was Shirley and she was fantastic!

She told me that a change of diet would help for starters.

I'm already a vegetarian and eat quite healthily, but she said I needed to eat every three hours to keep my blood sugar level balanced. And she was quite insistent that it was every three hours and not three hours and five minutes! Even a cracker as a snack mid morning or mid afternoon would be enough to keep my mood swings under control, providing I was eating proper meals at breakfast, lunch and supper.

She suggested I keep away from tea, coffee, sugar and dairy products, and recommended pasta instead of cakes for energy. She didn't tell me to keep off wheat, but I have read of some women whose PMS is exacerbated by a wheat allergy, though I don't seem to be one of them.

I made these dietary changes and quickly noticed the difference in the way I felt.

Having previously had premenstrual pain which prevented me from walking, the respite was like a breath of fresh air.

Shortly after making these dietary changes I went on a walking holiday to Cornwall. I had my period when I was there – and I didn't even notice it!

Shirley had told me that exercise would help a lot and, as well as walking, I played a lot of squash, which, she said, seemed good for me (though maybe not for everyone).

On the yoga side, she taught me specific exercises for the reproductive organs and I now do these, alone at home, for an hour every morning.

People ask how I manage to be so religious about my diet and yoga. All I can say is that if a doctor gave you a pill and told you it would save you from certain death, you would take it.

For me, sticking to my new diet and exercise routine is just as important because it brought my life back from the brink.

This chapter is packed with advice for the PMS sufferer who, like Louise, wishes to treat the problem without medical intervention. The suggestions here may also be recommended by a doctor treating you for PMS as an alternative to medication and they should also be considered alongside any medical treatment.

This chapter looks at how you can help yourself by means of:

- a change in diet
- a new exercise routine
- the use of vitamins and minerals
- learning to accept your PMS.

But, first, let us look at the role of nicotine, alcohol and caffeine in controlling PMS.

Caffeine is found in tea, coffee, cola, and chocolate as well as some painkillers and cough and cold medicines. It acts as a stimulant, and can cause anxiety, irritability, depression and nervousness. The link between caffeine and PMS is that the hormone oestrogen hinders the breakdown of caffeine. So, heavy consumption of caffeine drinks combined with high levels of oestrogen, where the high oestrogen theory appears to apply, seem likely to make symptoms such as anxiety and irritability much worse premenstrually.

Alcohol contains high levels of sugar, so consumption of it contributes to blood sugar mood swings. It is also a depressant of the central nervous system and can exacerbate insomnia, which also causes lethargy, clumsiness and depression.

Smoking should also be avoided as it can deplete the body's supplies of vitamin B_6, which is needed to counteract many of the symptoms of PMS.

So, the first rule, when taking self-help measures to treat your PMS, is to cut down on coffee and tea, alcohol and smoking.

Now for the rest of your new regime.

Diet

This may strike you as being rather strange, but many doctors still consider dietary treatment for PMS controversial! Many doctors are quite happy to prescribe antidepressants, tranquillizers and steroids, but ask whether changing one's eating habits will have any effect on relieving your symptoms and your doctor might cynically raise an eyebrow and say, 'Well, you can always try it, but I can't guarantee you'll have any success.'

What strikes me as being particularly odd about this reaction is that, while waiting to see the doctor about PMS, all kinds of 'healthy eating' pamphlets are displayed in the waiting room. Even if we visit the nurse for a new patients' check, we will be asked about our diet and advised to cut down on sugar, fatty meat and dairy products and eat more fruit, vegetables and fibre-rich foods. In fact, advice on healthy eating is often abundant – until we seek advice for treating our PMS.

Louise notes, 'Changing the way I ate made an instant difference to my PMS. But my doctor had never even mentioned diet!'

Of course, there are the enlightened few and, with luck, you will have a GP who recognizes that symptoms of PMS get worse when you skip meals and that shortages of some vitamins and minerals can also exacerbate the problem. However, you will make your GP's job (and yours) a lot easier if you have kept the charts described in Chapter 4, and noted the food and drink you have consumed around the time when you have suffered premenstrual symptoms.

In fact, the example I gave there of a typical day's eating and drinking makes pretty horrendous reading if you stop to consider the advice given about dairy products, refined carbohydrates, fatty meat, alcohol and caffeine. I listed, for breakfast, coffee, toast, butter and jam; for lunch, cheese and tomato sandwich; for supper, spaghetti bolognese and salad. And for fluids, I noted, during the morning, cups of coffee; at lunch, coke; during the afternoon, three cups of tea; in the evening, two glasses of red wine.

In this exanple, there's far too much caffeine and alcohol for starters. And the meals listed are high in meat and dairy fat and low in fibre.

Changing from a diet like this is difficult as old habits die hard, but a few simple changes can be introduced straight away. For example, instead of white bread, use wholemeal. Instead of butter use a polyunsaturated or olive oil-based spread. Instead of jam, have a banana. At lunchtime, have a wholemeal sandwich containing lean meat, instead of cheese, and salad. In the evening, use wholemeal pasta and a stir-fry vegetable sauce. Alternatively, if you are making bolognese sauce, fry the mince in a non-stick pan and drain off the fat before adding the meat to the other ingredients and use less of it and more vegetables. And, of course, make a big effort to cut down on the caffeine and alcohol. This is easier if it is done over a week or two, rather than overnight.

A diet to treat PMS needn't be a wacky one; it is just a sensible eating plan, which follows many of the basic rules in all those pamphlets in the doctor's waiting room. But, there is one important difference, which applies mainly to women experiencing symptoms premenstrually, and that is the advice Louise's yogic counsellor gave her: to eat regularly, every three hours.

Many women who suffer from PMS have found that their symptoms are exacerbated by low blood sugar levels. Keeping blood sugar levels at a safe level is therefore essential if treatment of PMS is to be successful.

The blood sugar level is the ratio of glucose to blood produced when carbohydrate foods (sugars, rice, potatoes, bread and cereals), are broken down in the digestive system. Glucose, the result of this breaking down process, passes into the bloodstream. Insulin is then released to help keep the amount of sugar in the blood at normal levels.

When long periods of time elapse between meals, or if meals are low in carbohydrate content, the blood sugar level falls. At this point, a spurt of adrenalin is released, allowing the blood sugar level to be topped up by some of the glucose from the body's stores. This process continues until more carbohydrate is consumed.

In women suffering from PMS, this release of adrenalin occurs more often. It has been found that attacks of aggression, panic, migraine, and so on are more likely to occur when there have been long intervals between meals or when meals have contained insufficient or no carbohydrate.

Blood sugar is affected not only by the amount of carbohydrate eaten, but also by the type. If your diet consists mainly of the refined carbohydrates (sugar, sweets and chocolates, cakes, white flour foods and polished rice), then the breakdown to glucose is much quicker than if your diet is rich in the unrefined carbohydrates (wholemeal bread, wholemeal flour, brown rice, high-fibre breakfast cereals, such as shredded wheat and porridge, pulses, jacket potatoes, fruit and vegetables).

The most sensible diet is a high-fibre diet, rich in foods from the group of unrefined carbohydrates as these will give you a sustained release of blood glucose, and, consequently, better regulation of your blood sugar levels.

Dr Michael Brush, a director of The Premenstrual Society, recommends that the following dietary guidelines be adopted to fight PMS:

- eat whole foods, not refined and processed 'fast' foods
- eat foods that are as fresh as possible (vegetables that are cooked should be cooked lightly, preferably steamed)
- all foods should be non-toxic for our bodies, that is, they should not contain artificial flavours, colours, preservatives or other food additives used to cosmetically enhance the food and increase sales – make a habit of reading the food labels when shopping and learn to decipher the additives
- within the guidelines, vary your diet – do not eat the same foods every day

- do not overeat – the goal should be undereating the right sorts of foods rather than overeating poorly balanced foods
- satisfying the craving for salt aggravates PMS, especially the bloating aspect of it, so resisting the urge to eat salty foods can reduce the severity of your symptoms
- satisfying the craving for sweets and sugary foods can result in hypoglycaemia-like attacks after the brief 'lift' given by the sugar has passed, as the symptoms of low blood sugar can accentuate the PMS symptoms of depression, agitation, fatigue, irritability and headaches, which are exactly like hypoglycaemic episodes
- prevent sweet cravings occurring by eating small and regular amounts of natural carbohydrates (fresh fruit, pulses, whole grains etc.) – the body was not designed to handle refined sugar in concentrated forms such as chocolates and cakes
- a diet that provides more protein than your body needs can cause severe deficiencies in many essential vitamins, including vitamin B_6 and niacin, and can actually drain important minerals, such as calcium, iron, zinc, phosphorus and magnesium, from the body (60 grams of protein a day should be sufficient)
- aim to include foods rich in essential fatty acids in your diet, such as seeds and nuts, grains and fish (especially oily fish such as mackerel), but avoid eating too many animal fats (saturated fats) such as are found in margarine, cheese and fatty meat.

You will not see the results of a change of diet overnight (it takes two to four months to achieve lasting results), but if you stray from the path of the good diet, the penalties may show up in a few weeks.

Your anti-PMS eating plan

Some pointers

A change of diet is nearly always daunting. It takes effort to change established habits and nobody likes the idea of being denied the foods they turn to for comfort.

Some organizations recommend major changes to the diet in order to treat PMS. These diets are usually based on the idea of *exclusion*, which is also the basis of diets that are used to treat allergies. An exclusion diet involves cropping the diet back so severely that you are left with only a handful of neutral basic ingredients, then gradually reintroducing foods to see which, if any, produce symptoms.

The exclusion diet is a very good way of identifying particular allergies and has been of benefit to thousands of people. However, it is also very drastic.

The following very straightforward, less drastic eating guidelines set by the National Association for Premenstrual Syndrome have proved just as effective, for many women, in treating PMS.

Looking at your own dietary charts, you will probably immediately identify easy changes you can make. Switching from white bread to wholemeal bread, for example, from white pasta to brown, from refined rice to brown rice and so on are all straightforward. Introduce the changes slowly and you will be amazed at how quickly you adapt to the new tastes. If you have ever given up taking sugar in your tea and coffee, you will know how sickly sweet and unbearable sugary drinks now taste. Converting from refined to unrefined foods is a very similar experience.

Because we are all different, with our own individual needs, it is impossible to lay down an eating plan that will suit everyone's requirements, and you are the only person who will be able to decide when you have arrived at the diet formula that best suits your own needs. Also, you are the only person who will know exactly how much to eat and when you need to eat your meals and snacks.

Very many women with PMS have a craving for sweet things and may binge on cakes and chocolates in the premenstrual phase. A good guide as to whether or not women with PMS are eating properly is to see if this symptom disappears.

A diet aimed at producing a sustained satisfactory blood glucose level throughout the whole month will, in itself, relieve many of the more severe symptoms of PMS and may, in fact, be all the 'treatment' that is required.

If progesterone supplements are needed, the diet must still be followed. Sudden adrenalin spurts are avoided by maintaining a steady blood glucose level.

This simple dietary regime is the key to successful treatment of PMS.

The basic plan

- *Breakfast (within half an hour of rising)*:
  - pure fruit juice or half a grapefruit
  - 5 tablespoons high-fibre breakfast cereal
  - 2 medium slices wholemeal bread, spread with polyunsaturated or low-fat spread
  - low- or reduced-sugar marmalade
  - tea or coffee with low-fat milk.
- *Mid morning*:
  - 1 digestive biscuit
  - tea or coffee with low-fat milk.
- *Midday or evening meal*:
  - lean meat or fish
  - 175g (6oz) jacket potato and a large helping of vegetables or salad
  - fresh fruit or tinned fruit in natural juice.
- *Mid afternoon*:
  - 1 digestive biscuit
  - tea or coffee with low-fat milk.
- *Evening or midday meal*:
  - vegetable soup
  - 2 slices wholemeal bread as a sandwich with meat or fish and salad
  - fresh fruit.
- *Bedtime or late evening*:
  - 4 high-fibre crackers
  - polyunsaturated margarine, small helping of cheese or lean meat, milky drink.

This basic plan gives you about 1400 calories each day, derived from high-fibre sources. A daily allowance of 600 ml (1 pt) of skimmed or semi-skimmed milk must be drunk daily to ensure an adequate calcium intake.

Varying your diet

To add variety to your diet, you can substitute one of the following – but no more than 3 to 4 portions of fruit per day should be eaten.

- *Cereals*:
  - 5 tablespoons All Bran
  - 5 tablespoons bran flakes
  - 4 tablespoons unsweetened muesli
  - 1 Shredded Wheat
  - 1 Weetabix
  - 6 tablespoons porridge
  - 1 medium slice of wholemeal bread
  - 75 g (3 oz) cooked brown rice
  - 4 low-calorie, high-fibre crispbreads
  - 75 g (3 oz) cooked wholemeal pasta
  - 1 digestive biscuit.
- *Fruit*:
  - 1 medium apple
  - 1 medium cooking apple
  - 1 large peach
  - 1 medium banana
  - 1 medium pear
  - 1 medium orange
  - 1 thick slice fresh pineapple
  - 2 large tangerines
  - 10 large grapes
  - 2 large dessert plums
  - 2 large stewed prunes
  - 175 g (6 oz) strawberries
  - 175 g (6 oz) raspberries.

All vegetables are relatively high in fibre, but the quantity you would need to eat in order to get a significant amount of carbohydrate is so large that it is impractical to supply your intake needs from this source alone.

Foods made with white flour, cakes, sweets, chocolate, biscuits and so on also contain carbohydrates, but they are not recommended as part of your normal diet. There is no reason why they should not be eaten as a treat, though.

Note that if you are going to be more energetic than usual – say, playing sports, gardening, spring cleaning – you should make sure you increase your intake of carbohydrates. Preferably eat before you take exercise, but, if this is difficult, eat afterwards.

How to watch your weight

At first glance you may think that this diet will cause you to put on weight as the carbohydrate content of the diet is being stressed, but this is not the case. Although you are increasing the amount of carbohydrate you consume from the unrefined sources, you are also being advised to cut down or cut out the sugars and sugary foods. You are also being advised to reduce your intake of fats. This combination will help you to lose weight slowly. But a careful watch should be kept on your weight as, by changing your eating habits, you may reduce your calorie intake to below what you need, thereby causing an unnecessary weight loss. So:

- weigh yourself once a week at the same time of day each time
- if you need to lose weight, decrease the quantity of carbo-hydrates, that is, take smaller portions of pasta, rice, baked potatoes, but do not compensate by eating more fatty foods
- if you do not need to lose weight, but discover that you are losing it anyway, increase the carbohydrate content of your meals.

Slimming on the PMS diet

Here is the 1000 calories a day eating plan.

- *Breakfast*:
  – pure fruit juice or half a grapefruit
  – 5 tablespoons high-fibre breakfast cereal
  – 1 medium slice of wholemeal bread, scraping of low-fat spread
  – low- or reduced-sugar marmalade
  – tea or coffee with low-fat milk.
- *Mid morning*:
  – 1 piece of fresh fruit
  – tea or coffee with low-fat milk.
- *Midday or evening meal*:
  – lean meat or fish
  – 175 g (6 oz) jacket potato
  – large helping vegetables or salad
  – 1 piece of fresh or tinned fruit in natural juice.
- *Mid afternoon*:
  – 1 piece of fresh fruit.
- *Evening or midday meal*:
  – vegetable soup
  – 1 slice of wholemeal bread or 3 Ryvita with meat or fish and salad
  – 1 piece of fresh fruit.
- *Bedtime or late evening snack*:
  – 2 high-fibre crackers with small helping of cheese or meat, etc.
  – milky drink.
- *Daily allowance*:
  – 600 ml (1 pt) skimmed milk
  – 25 g (1 oz) polyunsaturated margarine.

Here are some points to remember:

- if you are not used to a diet that is high in fibre, start gently when introducing it because if you don't, you'll suffer from bloating, flatulence, trapped wind and, possibly, stomach cramps

- when you change to this type of diet, you need to increase your fluid intake because otherwise you are likely to become constipated

- if you are on a medically prescribed diet for any reason, talk to your doctor and dietician to see if your present diet can be adapted to conform to the diet for PMS

- if you are a diabetic, you should already be on a high-fibre diet, bur do not change the prescribed carbohydrate portions without seeing your dietician first

- some people think they are getting all the right nutrients because they are taking supplements, but it is very important to be aware of the fact that whole, fresh foods, fresh fruit and vegetable juices and unpolluted water provide the foundation for a well-rounded diet

- in addition to avoiding processed foods, refined sugar and white flour foods, which have high salt contents, you should try to keep consumption of alcohol, caffeine, chocolate, nicotine and dairy products to a minimum – especially when you are experiencing PMS symptoms.

The Women's Nutritional Advisory Service goes one step further with its advice, providing women with individually tailored diets. The WNAS has identified a link between an allergy to wheat products and PMS in some women. While most of us can happily eat all the bread we like without our symptoms getting any worse, many have been helped by the WNAS's advice to avoid wheat products.

In Chapter 2, Carole told us how she discovered that depressive mood swings were a feature of her PMS. Here she describes how, after abandoning the antidepressants her doctor had prescribed, she tried the diet given to her by the WNAS.

The article in which another PMS sufferer described her mood swings went on to say that she had got rid of them – not with the help of pills or a psychiatrist – but by changing her diet!

I wrote to the WNAS who sent me a questionnaire asking me about my diet, lifestyle and moods. When I'd completed and returned it, they sent me a special diet plan which eliminated what seemed like nearly everything – coffee, tea, cheese, bread, cakes, chocolate and alcohol.

I dropped all these baddies overnight, which was perhaps a bit rash, as I experienced awful withdrawal symptoms for a week. Then I began to think, 'Is this really worth it?'

One morning at the end of that first week, I woke up feeling so rotten that I just got up, made the breakfast, then crawled back to bed – where I stayed all day and all night. But when I got up the following day, I felt fantastic! I hadn't felt that good in ages!

As with any diet, the first few months were the hardest. But the longer I was on it, the better I felt. Now, I have gradually reintroduced foods into my diet and can eat more or less anything I like – in moderation. I can actually control the way I feel with the things I eat.

When I look back, I can't believe how awful I used to feel. Today, I feel wonderful. I am confident, lively and energetic. And, best of all, those mood swings have gone . . . for good!

Exercise

If you do not exercise regularly, you can probably list the reasons preventing you from doing so . . . 'I'm too busy', 'There's nobody to look after the children', 'There aren't enough hours in the day', 'I don't want to be tied to fitness classes', even 'I get enough exercise running around after the kids and doing the housework'. These are all common excuses.

However, most of us, if we put our minds to it, can find time to do some form of exercise every day. Those who have squeezed exercise into their busy schedules and established a new routine very rarely look back. In fact, exercise can become such a pleasure that, once it is part of your daily routine, you will feel lost and irritable when you are prevented from doing it.

Apart from the physical activity involved in taking exercise, there is the fact that you are making time to do something for yourself, so it is as important that the exercise you choose gives you pleasure as it is that it improves your stamina and fitness.

Running around after children and hoovering the stairs do not constitute exercise. They involve muscle activity, but do not decrease depression or increase self-esteem. And for the treatment of PMS in particular, it is this self-nurturing aspect of exercise that is so vital.

Which type of exercise?

The ideal form of exercise should be:

- pleasurable, to boost self-esteem
- carried out daily at the same time every day – this way the body will come to rely on this regular release of tension
- last at least 30 minutes, uninterrupted.

For exercise to be helpful for PMS, it must include the commitment to take time out for oneself.

Plan your new exercise routine at the beginning of your cycle, just after your period starts, when you are feeling at your best (providing your period is not heavy or painful, in which case wait a few days for the flow to abate). It is a mistake to start something new when you are premenstrual as you will find it difficult to raise the necessary enthusiasm.

Try new forms of exercise as well as those you've always enjoyed. If you find yourself dreading a session at the swimming pool, think about an alternative that will give you pleasure. Disliking the activity you are pursuing defeats the object of exercise for the sake of PMS.

Swimming

Swimming is often quoted as the best form of exercise as it uses muscles you never knew you had! For the purpose of relieving PMS, it is less important to count the number of lengths you swim, or the speed at which you complete them, than it is to enjoy the experience.

Cycling

Cycling can be exhilarating, especially if you have access to pleasant countryside or a park to cycle in. This can be a great way to unwind and let your mind wander while releasing any pent-up tension by aerobic exertion.

Walking

Walking, at any pace, will release tension, as long as it is done for pleasure and not purely as a means of getting to work or rushing around the shops.

Other activities

Jogging, dancing, aerobics, horse riding and ball games can be included in your routine, but are less likely to be daily activities than swimming, cycling and walking.

Yoga

One of the best forms of exercise for the relief of PMS is yoga, which, in addition to relieving tension, has been found to normalize the hormonal imbalances and chemical changes in the blood that take place in PMS. This is achieved by means of a combination of posture, breathing and relaxation exercises.

Although there are many teach yourself-style books available on the subject of yoga, this is one form of exercise where it is really preferable to learn under supervision. You will be putting a lot of strain on certain parts of your body and incorrect posture or performing movements too jerkily can do more harm than good.

The very precise movements involved should always be practised under the guidance of a trained instructor, and it is usually easy to find local classes.

As well as promoting relaxation, yoga strengthens muscle tone and improves posture (bad posture can, in fact, have a detrimental effect on your health).

Posture and breathing exercise have a calming effect, physically and mentally. Some of the physical aspects of tension, such as tightness of the muscles, painful joints, shallow and inefficient breathing and a rapid heartbeat can be almost as troublesome during PMS as your outbursts of irritability. Learning how to control your breathing – in particular, how to breathe slowly and deeply – can relieve both types of symptoms. The lessening of tension in your muscles should help a lot, if muscular and joint aches and pains trouble you.

An upright and balanced posture, achieved with the practice of yoga, relieves a lot of the fatigue, lethargy and lower back pain experienced in PMS.

Sitting and lying techniques – particularly the seated forward bend, the backward seated bend (the bridge) and some of the twisting movements – are especially beneficial.

Ideally, you should aim to do 20 to 30 minutes of yoga per day, and to include in each daily session limbering, posture work, breathing and meditation or relaxation.

In a survey of 2600 people who do yoga by the British Yoga Biomedical Trust, 2000 were women who had suffered from PMS. Over 90 per cent of them reported that yoga had helped their PMS and that their symptoms continued to improve over a period of two years.

Vitamins and minerals

There are now numerous specially formulated combinations of vitamins and minerals (such as, Optivite, Magnesium OK) available for the treatment of PMS. Here we will look at why you may need to use supplements.

Vitamin B_6

As mentioned in the last chapter, your GP may advise, as a starting point in treating your PMS, the use of vitamin B_6 (also known as pyridoxine).

Vitamin B_6 is naturally present in your body, supplied in the foods you eat (especially wholemeal bread, red meat, liver, milk, eggs, yeast and rice polishings). But, in some people, this is not enough. They suffer a deficiency of vitamin B_6 that cannot be made up by a change in diet alone.

A deficiency of B_6 produces depression, bloating and acne, all common symptoms of PMS, and one theory about why the deficiency is so common among women with PMS is that high levels of oestrogen deplete supplies of this vitamin. High levels of vitamin B_6 are also vital for the healthy functioning of the hypothalamus, the control centre of the menstrual cycle.

Although vitamin B_6 is available in the form of tablets that can be bought over the counter from pharmacists, it is wise to discuss its use with your doctor before starting yourself on a course.

Dr Michael Brush recommends that vitamin B_6 treatment should be started three days before the onset of expected symptoms for maximum benefit.

As women vary greatly in the amount of B_6 they need to obtain a good response to treatment, you should start with two 20 mg tablets with breakfast, and two 20 mg tablets with your evening meal. If this dose does not appear to be having any effect, increase it to one 50 mg tablet twice daily. If it is still ineffectual, increase it to 60 or 75 mg twice daily. Each dose level should be tried for one or two menstrual cycles before moving up to a larger dose.

Once you have established the correct dose of B_6 for you, continue with it for six to eight months before attempting to reduce the dose. After that, if there are no problems, reduce the dose, step by step, by 25 to 50 mg, every four weeks. If your symptoms return, go back to the original, successful dose.

Note that vitamin B_6:

- is particularly useful for the relief of mood changes, breast discomfort and headaches
- should be balanced by adding other B vitamins to your daily intake (a standard vitamin B complex tablet will provide all you need)
- dosage may be too high and should be reduced if you experience an increase in headaches, nausea and restless sleep
- should always be taken with food to avoid stomach upsets
- has brought relief to thousands of PMS sufferers, but some

experts are still sceptical about its use and a group of doctors in the *New England Journal of Medicine* warned that taking vitamin B$_6$ in excessive doses can cause nerve damage.

Calcium and magnesium

In 1981, Dr Guy Abrahams found low levels of magnesium in many women suffering from PMS. The Women's Nutritional Advisory Service repeated his work by studying 105 women with PMS. The results showed that 45 of them had a magnesium deficiency.

Like calcium, levels of magnesium appear to fluctuate at different times in a woman's life. Requirements for both minerals increase greatly during pregnancy and breast feeding and a deficiency may exacerbate PMS after childbirth.

What is difficult to work out, however, is how much calcium and magnesium to take in supplement form to help PMS. The ratio of two parts calcium to one part magnesium (usually 500 mg to 250 mg) has traditionally been recommended to treat premenstrual and menstrual cramps. However:

- some women are only deficient in magnesium
- it is also thought that calcium depletes the body's supplies of magnesium.

Researchers have suggested that the ratio of calcium to magnesium be reversed. Dr Michelle Harrison, a leading authority on PMS, recommends, however, that doses should be varied according to the symptoms, so that for:

- premenstrual and menstrual cramps, but no other symptoms, two parts of calcium to one part magnesium should be taken
- PMS without cramps, one part calcium to two parts magnesium
- PMS cramps and other symptoms, equal amounts of calcium and magnesium.

Essential fatty acids

Evening primrose oil

A lack of EFAs can cause an abnormally sensitive reaction to even normal levels of prolactin, leading to an apparent excess of prolactin, and symptoms related to a progesterone and oestrogen imbalance.

By supplementing your natural levels of EFAs, you can relieve many of these symptoms.

Evening primrose oil is one of the richest sources of the EFA gamma-linolenic acid and this corrects underlying EFA deficiency at source by supplying what the body needs, thereby reaching the root of the problem. Several studies have shown evening primrose oil to be effective for symptoms such as breast tenderness and swelling as well as emotional symptoms.

Evening primrose oil is usually prepared in capsules of 0.5 g, to be taken three or four times daily throughout the month.

If the first month's treatment is not successful, increase dosage to six capsules daily during the second month, and maybe eight capsules daily during the third month if six do not appear to be enough.

Remember:

- always take evening primrose oil with food to avoid stomach upsets
- allergic reactions to evening primrose oil are rare, but do occur occasionally
- one word of warning: if you have *any* form of epilepsy, do *not* take evening primrose oil without consulting your doctor as there is some evidence that it can make the condition worse.

Learning to accept your PMS

PMS can make a big difference to your life. At home, at school and at work, you may feel hampered by tension, clumsiness and a general inability to cope. It helps if you can work out strategies to get you through these difficult times every month.

At home

Many women report that when they knew they had PMS, their families were the first to identify the monthly changes in them. As Nicky and Carole's stories illustrated in Chapter 2, it is possible to suffer with PMS and to be totally unaware of it. You may notice that your husband and children are getting on your nerves, that you feel under more pressure than usual and that arguments are erupting over silly little things, but you may not connect this with the time of month.

From inside the premenstrual woman, it appears that *everything* is going wrong – it is 'one of those days' and everybody seems to be against you. From the outside, where friends and relatives are standing, it is far easier to see the changes taking place. They see you become snappy, irrational and tearful. If someone points out that 'Mum's off again!', resist the urge to throw the nearest plate and, instead, try to look at the scene from their point of view.

If you're reading this and thinking, 'That's all very well, but I don't go out of my way to get annoyed with them, so what can I do to stop myself flying off the handle?', there *are* a few things you can do to make life easier for everyone at home.

- Avoid trigger situations. PMS is far worse when you are under pressure and minor incidents – getting behind with the housework, rushing to cook the evening meal – can be upsetting and make you feel as if life's on top of you when you are premenstrual. Especially if PMS makes you clumsy, causing you to trip over the hoover, break glasses instead of washing them and cut your fingers when you're chopping vegetables. Allow yourself more time for household chores and don't attempt to pack too many chores into one day. If premenstrually you feel tied to the house and housework, drop everything that is non-essential and leave more time for yourself.
- Pamper yourself, time hairdressing appointments and other things that make you feel good for your premenstrual phase.
- If you are forgetful, make lists to remind yourself of the things you have to do.

- Talk to your family about the way you feel and encourage them to help you. If the children are upset by the way you sound off at them premenstrually, perhaps they would agree to help with the housework and washing-up. If your husband or partner is used to you waking him with tea in the morning, perhaps he would agree to make you a cup of tea instead and allow you to wake up gently while he gets the children up for a few days every month. If your PMS is troubling the whole family, it has become a family problem and one the whole family has to overcome.

Fiona says, 'My present partner is totally understanding. He realizes it is not me but my PMS talking when I am forgetful and argumentative. He has even taught my three-year-old son to go to his room and leave me to it when I rant and rave!'

At work

The key to coping at work is to keep your day as stress-free as possible. This may seem difficult when you have little control over the amount of typing you will be asked to do, difficult clients you will have to speak to and numerous problems that all require your attention at once, but you can do it. Dr Caroline Shreeve advises:

- avoid driving if at all possible – make time to walk or get a lift to work
- hide tired or tearful eyes beneath dark glasses
- keep tissues and painkillers close at hand
- if you are in a position to organize your own working day, avoid scheduling 'heavy' meetings for your premenstrual phase
- try, if your job allows it, to 'get ahead of yourself' when you are *not* premenstrual, so you are not under too much pressure premenstrually
- make the most of your lunch hour to do something you enjoy – a walk in the park, a visit to a local library, a session at the public baths, a yoga class or a beauty treatment can all have the effect of making you feel better about yourself.

At school

If you are suffering from PMS in your teens, you are probably having to cope with the pressure of schoolwork and exams at the same time. So:

- get plenty of sleep to avoid lethargy and poor concentration in class
- talk to your best friend or your mother about any negative feelings you are experiencing because of depression – don't put up with feeling wretched just because you can't bring yourself to tell anyone how you feel
- if you don't feel like going out to parties, don't go – if being alone is what you really want, tell your friends that you need some time to be by yourself and if they suffer from PMS, too, they will know exactly how you feel
- if clumsiness is a problem, avoid dangerous sports pre-menstrually.

Counselling

For a lot of women, the supportive, understanding husband and family are a dream, not a reality.

Here are a few of the comments I got when I asked members of the National Association for Premenstrual Syndrome, 'How did your family cope with your PMS?'

They didn't.

They rejected me.

They made me feel I was a terrible mother.

They accused me of being greedy and self-indulgent for constantly snacking to keep up my blood sugar levels.

If, like these women, you are made to feel you have nobody to turn to, why not find a 'professional friend', a counsellor?

Counsellors, like your best friend, will listen, support and encourage you while you work out your problems and strategies for yourself. They will even help you to deal with your family by 'remote control counselling'!

Support groups

A common feeling among PMS sufferers is the sense that 'nobody understands'. This feeling of being the only person in the world with premenstrual difficulties can make you feel helpless to do anything about it.

A PMS support group is a place where you can share your feelings with women who know exactly what you're going through. It can also provide you with a list of emergency numbers to call for a bit of understanding when you are feeling angry and depressed premenstrually.

The National Association for Premenstrual Syndrome has local support groups all over Britain. If there is not a group near where you live, they will be able to advise you on setting one up.

If you are considering setting up a group, remember the following points:

- trying to take other people's problems on board can be stressful, so learn to balance your desire to help with the need to occasionally say 'No'
- your PMS will not be cured by becoming a group leader, but you will be just as helpful to others in your group if you can show them that you have come to terms with your PMS and learned to accept it and cope with it
- you will be subjected to some of the behaviour from other sufferers that your family puts up with when you are pre-menstrual – this should be an eye-opener and help you understand what your family is going through
- it's OK to laugh at your PMS – in fact, it is fantastically helpful if you can learn to see the funny side!

7

Alternative therapies

I have tried to stress throughout this book that there is no magic cure for PMS. What works for one woman, will be hopeless for another. But, by the same token, what is hopeless for your best friend may really do the trick for you. The point is to take time out to look at all the options. Try to be open-minded and patient (if your patience hasn't snapped completely!) and, eventually, you will find something that works for you.

As Joyce remarked, 'Vitamin B_6 has done the trick for me. I don't know if it's psychological, and I don't care. If the doctor told me I was taking Smarties I'd still carry on with them if I felt they were making me better!'

Personal experiences

Ruby took all the good advice about being open-minded and patient and tried just about every alternative therapy going. Here she sums up her experience.

My Chinese homeopathist gave me an infusion of herbs to make at home. They tasted awful, made my kitchen stink and cost a fortune . . . and I still had PMS!

Next I tried acupuncture, but, again, to no avail. My acupuncturist put a needle near my eye. It made me cry and because she didn't tell me she had removed it straight after insertion, I lay, in a terrified state, wondering what on earth was going to happen next.

Reflexology was relaxing, but the feeling wore off too quickly.

I decided that I could better deal with the stress if I learned to relax more, so I invested in some relaxation tapes. The problem is I only remember to use them when the stress is really bad and, by that time, I start to think that *nothing* will calm me down, so, to cut a long story short, they are getting very dusty.

I tried spiritual healing (nothing happened), meditation (I had the same problem sticking with this as with the tapes) and even hypnosis (which became very dangerous when I had problems coming out of my trance!).

I've used aromatherapy oils in a burner – lavender to keep me calm and eucalyptus to help me breathe. This is actually very relaxing – as long as I don't overdo the oils.

I've even had spiritual readings and looked into religion, but neither was of any use.

Do alternative therapies really have any benefit other than helping you to relax?

Like Ruby, a lot of people believe that alternative therapies can only help by helping you relax – and only then if you believe in them. But, Fiona's story shows that this need not be the case.

She had no faith whatsoever in homeopathy, but was at the end of her tether when she, quite reluctantly, took her friend's advice to give alternative medicine a try.

My GP had already tried everything she could. I hated the progesterone pessaries because they gave me thrush and, on four doses of 400 mg per day, I felt I was running out of places to put them! Oestradiol patches made me depressed. The Pill made me irrational. Danazol took me so low I couldn't be bothered with anything . . .

The only thing that did any good whatsoever was a prescription of steroid nasal spray, which worked by halting my cycle completely. But I knew I was going to have to come off that soon – it can only be used for six months, because of risks associated with osteoporosis – so I finally decided I had nothing more to lose by going to an alternative practitioner.

My friend had found a homeopath who specialized in women's problems, and she urged me to go to her.

I was very cynical. I have never understood how homeopathy can work or believed that it does.

But what immediately impressed me about Shaun, on my first consultation with her, was the attention she gave me.

She sat me down and got me to talk my life through with her, starting with my childhood.

When we got on to the specific problems I was experiencing premenstrually, she came up with a few remedies for me to try.

She was also, very unusually for a homeopath, willing to let me start on homeopathic remedies alongside the conventional medicine I was already taking, and this meant I could ease myself off the nasal spray with the knowledge that I was being cushioned by a new treatment.

To be perfectly honest, though, none of Shaun's remedies seemed to do me any good for the first few months – in fact, most of them made me feel an awful lot worse! But I continued to see Shaun every week, because here was someone who was actually willing to listen to me and to try to help me.

She took on board the fact that PMS was making my life extremely difficult and was also honest enough to admit that she hadn't found the right treatment for me yet.

Money wasn't an issue, because I was fortunate enough to be able to see Shaun very cheaply through my local Well Woman Clinic. So I knew that she certainly wasn't spinning out my treatment for the sake of a decent profit.

I suppose I stuck with her because she had gained my trust and confidence. And because she was as keen as I was to get my PMS sorted out.

After about three or four weeks, she suggested I might also try aromatherapy. One of my problems was poor self-image. Premenstrually I hated myself so much I had frequently tried to cut and hurt myself.

Shaun had the idea that aromatherapy would restore my self-esteem and make me feel good about my body again.

The main benefit, I feel, is the pure and luxurious self-indulgence of a massage. Premenstrually you need time to yourself, to feel important, and an aromatherapy back massage provides that. It is nothing but absolutely nice!

Meanwhile Shaun and I persevered with trying to find a remedy that would treat my mood swings. Most of them continued to be ineffectual and, after six months of trying, I was beginning to despair of ever getting the treatment I needed.

Then, finally, Shaun gave me a remedy that produced no emotional symptoms, but, instead, I suffered the most terrible fever! I had never felt so cold in all my life. I was convinced I was going to die. And, not making the connection with homeopathy, I called my GP out a couple of times.

When I told Shaun at my next consultation with her, she explained that what I had experienced was the 'classic picture' of the remedy I had taken and I'd probably taken too much of it.

She was pleased when the emotional symptoms subsided and physical symptoms took over. She said it showed that my body was cleansing itself of all the old anger and violence and also that I was no longer seeing my body as something separate, which I had previously hated and wanted to destroy.

Since then, she has established the correct dose for me and, when I wake up premenstrually and feel the emotions building up, I know I can take my remedy and be immediately calmed down.

Barbara had turned to acupuncture at the age of 19, after having no joy with the GP she'd been seeing about the neck and back tension that were hampering her studies at University.

I eventually decided to spend all the spare cash I had on something that would ease my pain and allow me to get through my exams.

At the time, PMS was not an issue and I don't think the tension was related to PMS, because it wasn't cyclical – I had it nearly all the time.

But then, about three years ago, I realized that premenstrually I was becoming very aggressive. For about three or four days before my period, I would argue and, worst of all, pick on people for very little reason.

I didn't go around picking on people willy nilly. Instead, I would target somebody and make their life a misery.

Once I gave my mother an unwarranted earful of abuse for things that had happened in my childhood that I'd magnified out of all proportion. Several times I had a go at my partner for all his shortcomings – from his side it must have seemed extremely hurtful and unfair that, suddenly, I was having a go about everything I disliked about him, when he had done nothing to invite such an attack.

But, worst of all, I started shouting at a complete stranger in a supermarket when he had to deal with my enquiry after I took some goods back.

I realized then that I was getting totally out of control and needed help.

I was still seeing my acupuncturist, who combined acupuncture treatment with osteopathy, fairly regularly for back and neck tension, so I mentioned my aggressive outbursts to him.

He said that a lot of it was deep-seated, from way back in my childhood, and that it only manifested itself when my hormonal levels were changing premenstrually.

Together we worked out that my premenstrual symptoms were a general barometer of other problems in my life – and definitely my aggression seemed to be worse premenstrually when I had a lot of stress on.

My acupuncturist was able to relieve a lot of this stress through a technique he calls 'windows to the sky', which is the release of past aggression and negativity, and I found this helped a great deal.

But, just as helpful was the fact that I had identified the underlying aggression and problems that I could then take to a counsellor.

Partly with my acupuncturist's help, and partly through my own determination to bring my problem under control, I have now got rid of all the aggression I used to experience premenstrually.

I am still more sensitive to disappointment than I am during the rest of my cycle and more negative premenstrually than I am mid cycle, but I can deal with it and, most importantly, I don't let it upset my relationships with other people.

Why try alternative medicine?

If you have always got on well with your GP, have been able to take your time in talking your problems over with him or her and have found most of the treatments prescribed successful (and have been happy with the medication prescribed), then you have very little reason to try alternative medicine. Better the devil you know, as the saying goes.

But, sadly, many women complain that they do not get a fully sympathetic service from their doctor. GPs are busy people and they don't always have the time to listen to you. Surveys have revealed that women, in particular, come away from consultations feeling frustrated and dissatisfied.

Part of this dissatisfaction is due to the amount of time women are forced to spend with their doctors. Our basic biological functions – menstruation, pregnancy, childbirth and menopause – all involve trips to the doctor and, during our reproductive years we visit the doctor twice as often as men.

The difficulties we experience with our doctors – feeling we are not being taken seriously and worrying about how to get the full message of our symptoms across in the alloted time, when, very often our GP is looking at his or her watch, and still writing up the last patient's notes when we are talking – only partly explain the increased interest in unorthodox medicine.

There is also the fact that so many modern drugs produce unpleasant side-effects. Everyone worries about another thalidomide – and none of us wants to think that the wonder drug we are on is one day going to be a front-page newspaper scandal.

The realization that modern medicine *doesn't* have all the answers is good news in some respects because it means we have all become more open to the other options available.

While nobody can pretend that alternative medicine will work miracles, it has done wonders for thousands of people who now swear by it. And it can work very well in the treatment of PMS.

All alternative therapies aim to treat you as a whole person. This means that, instead of treating an individual symptom on its own, the alternative practitioner will want to know all about you – about your work, your home, your family, the foods you eat, the activities you do. . . . The picture of you that he or she forms from the information you give is particularly useful in the treatment of a condition like PMS where so many different factors are involved.

In many ways, alternative therapies can be seen as a luxury and a self-indulgence. They give you the chance to talk about yourself and nothing but yourself, provide you with a captive audience and, like all luxuries, alternative medicine rarely comes cheap.

Don't let the cost put you off, though. There are women's natural health centres all round Britain that offer alternative therapies at a discounted rate for low-income families. And more and more orthodox doctors are coming round to the idea of offering some kind of alternative medicine from their practice.

Finding a therapist

Most alternative therapists have to undergo lengthy training before they can practise, but the main criticism levied against them remains that practitioners are not adequately regulated. So how do you find a reputable practitioner?

It is impossible to give guidelines that will *guarantee* that you find a good practitioner, but the following tips are worth bearing in mind when you are starting to look around:

- ask friends to recommend someone they have found helpful
- check that the practitioner is registerd with a professional body, such as the Society of Homeopaths or the British Acupuncture Association and Register
- ask your doctor if he or she can recommend anyone
- before making an appointment, ask the practitioner if he or she has previously treated women with PMS and, if so, what success he or she has had.

- go for a practitioner who operates a sliding scale of fees and find out before your first appointment how much you can expect to pay
- don't expect miracles or an instant cure – most alternative therapies are gentle and take a while to work.

Which therapy?

Acupuncture

What is it?

Of all the alternative therapies, acupuncture has gained the most surprising amount of respect in the medical world. Once viewed with complete distrust, it is now attracting quite serious interest and has been used by dentists and surgeons for anaesthetic purposes.

Your acupuncturist will take a detailed history from you, asking about your emotions and background as well as your specific symptoms.

He or she will then examine you to see where any imbalances lie as acupuncture is based on the theory that our health is governed by a flow of energy known as *ch'i*, which travels through our bodies from one organ to another. A blockage or imbalance in this flow of energy can bring about ill-health.

On the basis of the diagnosis the acupuncturist will place needles in selected points on invisible lines called meridians, with a view to unblocking the flow of *ch'i* to restore balance and harmony in the body.

How can it help PMS?

Because acupuncture treats each patient as an individual, two women presenting with the same set of PMS symptoms are likely to receive quite different treatment. Acupuncturists compare their diagnosis procedure to peeling off the skins of an onion until the core of the problem is found. Your therapist will base the treatment on this underlying cause.

The treatment chosen will also depend very much on the school of acupuncture your practitioner follows.

Some acupuncturists recognize a condition known as 'empty blood', which can lead to period problems and depression. By stimulating the points that influence the blood, in order to increase its production and flow, acupuncturists hope to bring relief to PMS.

Energy blocks in the channels known as the Governor Vessel and the Conception Vessel are particularly common in conditions of PMS. When they are unblocked, you should, according to acupuncturists, experience a normal hormonal cycle, free of particularly troublesome symptoms.

You may be treated separately for specific symptoms, such as migraine, backache, insomnia or addictions.

There is also speculation that acupuncture affects neurotransmitter levels, which have a direct effect on the hypothalamus, the control centre of the menstrual cycle.

Homeopathy

What is it?

Homeopathy works on the principle of 'like treating like'. Patients are treated with remedies that, in their crudest form, would bring on the very symptoms they are experiencing. So, instead of giving an insomniac something to produce artificial sleep, the homeopath will give his or her patient a minute dose of a substance that (in large doses) would cause a healthy person to become sleepless. Surprisingly, this will enable the sleepless person to sleep naturally and, because the dose is so minuscule, there are no side-effects.

Homeopathic remedies work by stimulating the body's own natural healing power and practitioners believe very strongly in the need to treat each patient as a separate individual. What works wonders for one person suffering from headaches may do nothing whatsoever for another patient complaining of the same problem. So, although homeopathic remedies are available from healthfood shops and chemists, the best advice is to make an appointment to see a homeopathic practitioner.

He or she will be looking very closely into the background of your complaint and although a lot of the questions asked are about your past, even your mother and grandmother, and may seem quite irrelevant, the practitioner will be using these details to form a picture of your state of health, and this picture will help him or her to identify the most accurate remedy for you.

Patients sometimes experience physical symptoms, such as colds or rashes, after starting on a course of homeopathic treatment, but, if you do experience something like this, it should not last long and is just the result of the body's spring cleaning process (however you should contact your practitioner immediately if your symptoms become worrying or very troublesome).

How can it help PMS?

Specific remedies for PMS include:

- calc carb, for tender breasts
- graphites, for weight gain
- lycopodium, for depression
- nat mur, for irritability
- nux vom, for argumentativeness
- pulsatilla, for weepiness
- sepia, for mood swings.

However, homeopathic practitioners believe that true PMS is more than just feeling rotten in the week before your period starts. As all disease and illness has an underlying cause, it is important to identify the root of the problem and treat it. If a woman becomes sad, angry or violent during her premenstrual week, she is manifesting feelings that may always be present, but which she normally manages to suppress or somehow ignore.

These feelings may be unresolved anxieties from as far back as childhood, so your practitioner will be looking at your background – especially family problems or childhood insecurities – and, on a physical level, he or she may even ask about your mother and grandmother's experiences of menstruation (if you are able to shed any light on this) for signs of family susceptibility to menstrual problems.

He or she will also want to know about your cycle and about the type and flow of your monthly periods. Do you experience physical symptoms, such as cramping as well as emotional symptoms like sadness, for example?

Very often one remedy, such as sepia, the classic remedy for PMS, will treat the problem, but you may need to combine homeopathy with other therapies, such as counselling or aromatherapy, which will help to boost your self-esteem.

Herbalism

What is it?

Although herbalism has been around for a very long time, it has only recently gained popularity. One of the main attractions is that, unlike orthodox medicines, which are often harsh and may have potentially harmful side-effects, herbal remedies are very gentle, but also very effective.

Like the homeopath and acupuncturist, the herbalist will be looking at you as an individual before prescribing a remedy and so your first consultation will include a long discussion about your past medical history as well as the routine tests on blood pressure, urine and haemoglobin that you would expect if you were visiting a conventional doctor.

Treatments are normally in the form of syrups or tinctures, but, occasionally, you will be given dried herbs to make up as an infusion (tea). Poultices, ointments and lotions may also be prescribed for external use.

How can it help PMS?

The Medical Herbalist Elisabeth Brooke believes that the liver has a large part to play in controlling our PMS. She claims that as everything from the air we breathe to the hormones we secrete passes through the liver, where it is sorted into good and bad groups and redistributed around the body as necessary, there must be a fault in the liver that is preventing the correct breakdown and redirection of hormones from taking place.

The fault is probably due to the excess of toxins – from

pollutants, caffeine, drugs and food additives – that we have to contend with daily and which have worn our poor livers out.

It follows, therefore, that by reducing your intake of poisons, you will take some of the strain off your liver and it will be better equipped to cope with the monthly shift in hormone levels.

Cutting down on alcohol, nicotine and food additives will all help considerably.

Your herbalist will also prescribe herbal remedies, such as marigold, dandelion and gentian root, to restore the balance within your liver, and vitex and lady's mantle, to balance your hormones. False unicorn root and skullcap will work as relaxants.

Herbs should be taken throughout the menstrual cycle for at least two cycles for a clear effect to be seen.

For mild PMS, a mixture of marigold and lady's mantle will usually be effective, while for severe or long-standing PMS, chaste berry and dandelion root, or gentian root and false unicorn root are usually helpful.

For over-the-counter remedies, try scullcap and valerian tablets to ease tension, dandelion to help with fluid retention or vitex agnus castus (Chase tree), a progesterone-like herb that helps improve pituitary function and hormone levels.

Naturopathy

What is it?

The naturopath believes illness is a sign that the body is trying to get itself back to normal, so, instead of suppressing the symptoms of your illness, your practitioner will encourage them. If you have a temperature, for example, a naturopath will use techniques to encourage your body to sweat as a way of getting rid of accumulated waste products.

However, most naturopaths encourage a healthy diet and lifestyle as a way of preventing illness from occurring in the first place.

Disease can be divided into three groups according to naturopathy. These are:

- *chemical* where nutritional deficiencies or excesses lead to poor functioning of the lungs, kidneys, bowels and circulation
- *mechanical* where poor posture, stiff muscles and joints lead to problems with the functioning of the nervous system and the musculoskeletal system
- *psychological* where stress leads to problems affecting the whole body.

The idea of naturopathy is to get rid of the body's poisons so that the body is in the best position to heal itself.

Treatment includes:

- fasting, to rid the body of waste (which should only be done under supervision)
- a diet of raw foods and unrefined carbohydrates and a small amount of protein
- hydrotherapy, with applications of hot and cold water in the form of baths, ice packs, compresses, sprays and douches
- structural adjustments, by means of osteopathy, chiropractic, exercise and realignment techniques, such as the Alexander Technique
- natural hygiene, which encourages a positive approach to life.

How can it help PMS?

Naturopathy encompasses much of the general self-help advice for PMS. And we have already seen how diet and exercise, relaxation and better posture can, in many cases, lessen the burden of PMS.

Shiatsu

What is it?

Shiatsu is based on the same principles as acupuncture but, instead of using needles, practitioners use finger, thumb, elbow and even knee pressure to stimulate the body's vital energy flow.

Physically this has the effect of helping to release toxins and deep-seated tension from the muscles, as well as stimulating the hormone system.

It is also a deeply relaxing therapy, which encourages patients to get in touch with their natural healing abilities.

In order to gain the most benefit from a Shiatsu treatment, you should follow these basic guidelines:

- don't eat heavy meals or drink alcohol on the day of treatment, but have a light meal at least one hour before your session
- do not take a long hot bath on the day of treatment
- wear loose, comfortable clothing, preferably cotton, such as a jogging suit (you will usually remain fully clothed during the session, which takes place on a padded surface at floor level)
- let your practitioner know of any medication you are currently taking.

After a shiatsu session, you will probably feel invigorated yet relaxed. Sometimes the first benefits to occur do not improve the main complaint but, rather, your overall health.

Duration of treatment varies between patients. Most people are torn between their desire to get better and the reluctance to give up old behavioural patterns that reinforce sickness. You will only begin to feel completely better when you are able to give yourself over to a new and healthy lifestyle.

Some patients experience temporary healing reactions as toxins and negative emotions are released. These may take the form of a headache or flu-like symptoms for 24 hours. In such cases, contact your therapist.

How can it help PMS?

Like the other alternative therapies mentioned in this chapter, treatment will involve advice on diet, exercise and lifestyle, from which you will learn how to look after yourself generally. This, in turn, leads to improved self-esteem and peace of mind for the patient.

Shiatsu practitioners also believe that the reproductive system is influenced by internal body rhythms, regulated by the hormonal system and blood circulation, and that imbalances can manifest themselves as menstrual and premenstrual problems.

A better diet and lifestyle will help to restore the balance, but your practitioner will also use techniques to regulate the *ch'i* energy and blood in the internal organs. In particular, he or she will concentrate on the liver, which stores the blood and smooths *ch'i* flow, and the spleen, the function of which is to prevent haemorrhage.

He or she may also suggest:

- treating the stomach and small intestine channels and points on the liver and spleen channels to relieve period pains
- tonifying the points on the bladder channel in the mid and lower back to relieve pain and dizziness after a period
- shiatsu to the feet, big toe and lower belly to lessen heavy menstruation
- calming the mind by calming the heart and spleen channels.

Some shiatsu exercises, such as the following, can be done at home as part of your self-help programme, although it is best to get advice from a practitioner as to exactly how to do this so that you are sure you are doing the right thing:

- applying gentle finger pressure at the nape of the neck helps to rebalance PMS, depression and headaches caused by hormone imbalances
- gentle pressure applied to the indentations at the top of the eye sockets will soothe away headaches and stress
- swollen, sore breasts will benefit from gentle massage to the indentation to the side of the back of the neck
- to ease premenstrual bloating, apply firm pressure to the back of the ankle
- to ease stomach cramps, shiatsu practitioners recommend heating two cupfuls of sea salt in a dry skillet, sprinkling the hot salt on half a folded towel and folding the other half of the towel over the salt to create a sandwich, lying down, relaxing and applying the warm salt towel to your stomach. The warmth and the energy-drawing effect of the sea salt will ease

away the cramp, and is said to work much better than a hot water bottle.

Chiropractic

What is it?

Chiropratic involves manipulating and adjusting the spine and other joints and is based on the idea that the spine protects the spinal cord, so if the spine is not in proper alignment, it interferes with the nerve supply, causing the body not to function properly.

Your chiropractor will take a full case history and may use X-rays to help with diagnosis. Treatment consists of thrusting directly on certain bones (a process called adjustment) with a view to encouraging them to return to their correct positions.

How can it help PMS?

This kind of pressure on the body can result in the surfacing of hidden emotions and repressed feelings, which many alternative practitioners believe play a leading role in PMS. Once these feelings are freed, they can be dealt with and this should have the effect of easing much of the tension experienced in PMS.

Other therapies

Other hands-on therapies, such as osteopathy, acupressure, aromatherapy, foot reflexology and therapeutic touch are also beneficial to sufferers of PMS. But the general advice for all alternative therapies is to try to find a practitioner who is happy to let you combine therapies. You may find, like Fiona, that a combination of homeopathy with hands-on aromatherapy or, like Barbara, that acupuncture combined with osteopathy works best for you.

8

The up-side of PMS

'*What* up-side of PMS?', I hear you gasp. 'How can anything *good* come out of something so utterly *bad*?'

The up-side of PMS is a grey area, but it cannot be dismissed.

Premenstrual women are very sensitive to emotions, sounds, smells. Women who are creative – artists, writers and musicians – report that, premenstrually, they experience an upsurge in ideas. They dream more, have more creative ideas and are more easily inspired. The majority of women, however, do not have this creative bent and, for them, the negative symptoms of PMS tend to overshadow anything positive they may experience.

However, a study of 102 woman at Canadian Well Woman Clinics in 1989 revealed that seven out of ten women experienced at least *one* positive symptom in their premenstrual phase. Among these were:

- more energy – 18 per cent
- more imaginative ideas at work – 11 per cent
- increased confidence – 6 per cent
- increased enjoyment of sex – 31 per cent
- fuller, more attractive breasts – and therefore increased self-esteem – 20 per cent
- a tendency to get things done – 29 per cent.

Critics of PMS argue that the reason so little is made of positive symptoms is that women are always asked about how depressed they feel prior to a period and never about how creative they are at this time, but then doctors have little reason to treat women who feel happy, buoyant and creative!

Even if you are not one of the lucky few women who report positive symptoms, there may be an up-side to your own experience that you can harness.

Use your premenstrual phase to do the following:

- *Sort your life out* Theresa has suffered from PMS since her early thirties.

  One of my main problems used to be that I would react angrily and impulsively if something happened to upset me. If my landlord wrote to tell me he was raising my rent, and his letter arrived when I was premenstrual, I would be straight on the phone telling him what I thought of him.

  The problem, as I soon learned, was that I was creating storms when I was premenstrual that would then have repercussions for the rest of the month. Having overreacted to my landlord, it was then very difficult to go back and make amends when, in my more rational weeks, I realized there was a more productive way of handling the issue.

  Now, I know my cycle by heart. I can tell when my blood is boiling premenstrually, but, instead of letting my temper erupt, my strategy for dealing with other people is to take a deep breath and put the problem aside for the following week.

  I find that any problems that have been niggling at the back of my mind tend to come to the fore when I am premenstrual. And this is a good time to capitalize on the feeling of urgency to get things done.

  For example, problems at work might wash over me during the three weeks when I am *not* premenstrual, but the week before my period I will have a sudden burst of desire to change my job. That is the week I will send off for application forms and think about the alternatives available to me.

  To me, this is a positive aspect of PMS. Because, without that monthly surge of troubleshooting, my life would be stagnant. We all need times like this to spring-clean our lives, sort out our problems and move ourselves on.

- *Make the most of your sexuality* Sarah says that her own experience of PMS has made her very much more aware of her own menstrual cycle and, from the pattern that has developed, she knows exactly when in the month she will want sex – and when she certainly does not.

The week before my period I am low and lethargic and have no interest in sex. But I am not completely negative about it because, during this time, I know I have something to look forward to. The week of my period is a very energetic, elated and sexual time for me.

In a way I have come to see this time as death and rebirth. I have to go down, premenstrually, in order to fully appreciate the high I experience during my period.

I have two sexual peaks during my cycle. The first is during my period, when I am very animal-like in my desire for sex. The second is around ovulation, when I am on more of an emotional high. These two peaks bring about completely different types of sexual experience and I relish this variety.

I believe very strongly that women should go with their cycle and not be pressured by their partners to have sex when, for them, it is not the right time.

For centuries, women have fallen in with men's sexual needs and I think that, by doing this, and by having sex when we do not want it, we risk throwing our cycles out completely. That can mean having sex when you don't want it, and subsequently not wanting it when, naturally, you should.

I am single right now, but my last partner was very aware of the fact that my sexuality is biologically controlled. I think he would have preferred it to be romantically controlled, but he agreed, unusually for a man, that it was better for men to fit in with women than the other way around.

Because we talked about my sexuality, and he understood that my needs were governed by my hormones, he never took it as a personal insult that I didn't want sex when maybe he did. And this took off a lot of the pressure that other couples experience.

Once you realize you can control your sex life, it is really not difficult to improve it. A lot of couples' problems come about because they are compromising their own sexual desires to fit in with their partner. I will never do that, and I make that clear at the start of any relationship so there are no misunderstandings.

- *Appreciate the variety and depth of your personality* PMS makes Mary so weepy, negative and incapable, that she now schedules her life around it.

During that week I can get nothing done, so I arrange as little as possible and, really, take the week off.

The rest of the month, I am extremely energetic. I am a very forward person and people often ask, 'Where do you get all that vitality?'

It's taken me a while to appreciate that, in spite of my PMS, or perhaps because of it, I have a bright side to my personality as well as a dark side.

As much as I hate PMS, I do feel it has contributed to my life. The thought of getting rid of it completely has become easier to accept as I've progressed with my treatment. But if, several years ago, someone had said, 'Press this button and your PMS will go away forever', I would have replied, 'Can't I get rid of it one bit at a time?' PMS was a part of me and I was actually scared of losing it completely!

I've had a lot of misplaced psychotherapy because of my symptoms, but this has opened my eyes and I now find 'me' an exciting, complex person.

- *Make the most of your dreams* Psychologists have found that, premenstrually, women's dreams are either very sexual or very aggressive. Taking an interest in your premenstrual dreams, and recording them in a diary, will increase your understanding of the depths of your character and should help boost your self-esteem. For example, if you cope well in a dream situation that you would not have been able to deal with in real life, take this as a sign that you do have the capacity to cope, even though you may not previously have been aware of it. Fiona has the following experience.

Premenstrually I am often awake in the middle of the night and by morning, I feel tired and exhausted – as if I haven't slept at all.

My boyfriend says that I sit bolt upright, screaming. I am

totally unaware of this as it takes place in my sleep. These episodes are known as 'night terrors' and I only experience them premenstrually.

I also have very violent dreams before my period and these I *do* remember. Usually they start with an argument with my parents or step-parents and, by the end of the dream, they are trying to kill me. Many times I've woken in a sweat when one of them has been holding me under water.

They do not appear to be at all productive, but, through these dreams, I have come to terms with the fact that I do not like my parents. I used to feel a lot of guilt about this. Now I feel I have dealt with the situation. I still see my Mum and Dad, but I do not expect anything from the relationship. In my own situation it has been helpful for me to reach this stage.

With my homeopathist, Shaun, I have worked out that I have a lot of unresolved anxieties from childhood. And I think these dreams are a way of releasing some of the aggression I still feel about that premenstrually.

It has been said that men can experience PMS-like symptoms if they are deprived of sleep for a few nights – and researchers have pointed out that it is not so much the sleep deprivation that causes lethargy, irritability and clumsiness, but the fact that one is deprived of dreams.

Ernest Hartman, a sleep expert, found that premenstrual symptoms were worse when women hadn't been able to sleep well and improved when they had slept more than usual. This may mean that, in some cases, women who report little or no PMS have a very active dream life during this phase of their cycle. But how can you improve your dream life? If insomnia, or restlessness at night, is a feature of your PMS, look at ways of improving the quality of your sleep. Sleeping tablets can get you off to sleep, but do not promote a relaxing and satisfying night's sleep. Use some of the relaxation techniques (yoga, and alternative therapies) described in this book. Cut down on caffeine, especially after midday, and avoid alcohol, which is a stimulant. Take exercise during the day as inertia will contribute to a restless night. Also, stick to a routine – go to bed at the same time every night and set your alarm clock for the same time in the morning. Studies have shown that many people with insomnia sleep much more than they think they do, but they tend to wake up a lot during the night. Your sleep should be measured by quality, not quantity. Look forward to your dreams and plan ahead for your nocturnal adventures. Once you have a regular record of your dreams, you will be able to analyse them and work out for yourself whether or not they relate to your PMS.

- *Learn to look after yourself.* This book has been all about learning to look after yourself. Bad diet, lack of exercise, stress and the inability to relax will take their toll on anyone. Even if your particular set of symptoms respond only to drastic treatment, PMS is as good an excuse as any to take your general health by the horns and give it a good shake up!

Useful addresses

National Association for Premenstrual Syndrome (NAPS)
PO Box 72
Sevenoaks
Kent
TN13 1QX
01732 459378

Women's Nutritional Advisory Service
PO Box 268
Lewes
East Sussex
BN7 2QN
01273 487366

Premenstrual Society (PREMSOC)
PO Box 102
London
SE1 7ES

British Homoeopathic Association (BHA)
27a Devonshire Street
London
W1N 1RJ
0171 935 2163

British Acupuncture Association and Register
34 Alderney Street
London
SW1V 4EU
0171 834 1012

Natural Medicines Society (NMS)
Edith Lewis House
Back Lane
Ilkeston
Derby
DE7 8EJ
01602 329454

Yoga For Health Foundation
Ickwell Bury
Biggleswade
Bedfordshire
SG18 9EF
01767 627271

Further reading

Dalton, Katharina, *Once a Month: Menstrual Syndrome, Its Causes and Consequences*. Fontana, 1983.

Harrison, Dr Michelle, *Self-help with Premenstrual Syndrome*. Optima, 1991.

Stewart, Maryon and Abraham, Guy, *Beat PMS through Diet*. Vermilion, 1994.

Shreeve, Dr Caroline, *Premenstrual Syndrome: How to Overcome the Monthly Blues*. Piccadilly, 1994.

Stewart, Maryon, *Beat Sugar Craving: The Revolutionary 4 Week Diet*. Vermilion, 1992.

Index